INVINCIBILITY IN THE FACE OF PROSTATE CANCER : COMING OUT THE OTHER SIDE

WE CANNOT CHANGE THE CARDS WE ARE DEALT, JUST HOW WE PLAY THE HAND.

ALFRED SAMUELS

First published in the United Kingdom in 2015 by
The Cloister House Press
ISBN 978-1-909465-43-5

Dedications

My children, my Inspiration and my love

Grace & Joshua, your love and affection is ever-flowing

My brother, Kelly, the truest of brothers

My sisters Valentina and Doreen - God worked His ways through you to me

My friends "Forever" you know who you are

The Almighty; in Him all is possible, Nothing takes him by surprise, even "cancer"

The late Gordon Holt - Never a truer dear friend. R.I.P

For all cancer sufferers and survivors, wherever you may be – "May this time of suffering become something beautiful in your life also."

"You have taken a hit. Life has knocked you down, but you are not knocked out. You have more going for you than you realize. Others might laugh and say you are through. But they do not know you like that. You have the ability to pull victory from the jaws of defeat! Now is the time for you to gather your wits; clear your head and mind; and dig down deep.

Resolve to unleash your creative energy, unstoppable attitude and resourcefulness. This is your time and your moment to prove to yourself and everyone else who you really are. You have the power to change your circumstances; change your finances; love again; rebuild relationships; and create your own job or business. You have the power to open the doors of possibility and move your life forward. You have the power within you because you have something special. You have GREATNESS within you!"

Les Brown
Motivational Speaker

TABLE OF CONTENTS

Acknowledgements

Mount Vernon Cancer Treatment Centre,
Mount Vernon Hospital.
Hertfordshire U.K

Consultant Oncologist
Dr Peter Ostler, MBBS, MRCP, FRCR,

Oncologist
Dr Shiv Gayadeen, MBBS, MRCP, FRCR,

Specialist Research Nurse
Elaine Lousley

The Nursing Staff on the Marie Curie Wing

Dr. M. Rodgers

PREFACE

My name is Alfred Samuels, and I am 57 years old. This is a true and continuing personal story of my struggle against advanced metastatic prostate cancer. I hope this book will educate and empower others in a similar situation and assist cancer researchers seeking to understand the detailed, personal and debilitating physical feelings of a cancer sufferer. Before diagnosis, I weighed 121 kg and stood at 6 ft with a large physical build.

IT IS VIRTUALLY impossible to pick up any nationally syndicated UK newspaper or watch any broadcast or cable channel without seeing the spectre of "cancer" raised. In the case of prostate cancer, it is the second leading cause of mortality in the western world. It is the single most common non-cutaneous malignancy in the United States, with 241,740 occurrences and 28,170, deaths in 2012 alone. Every year, 35,000 men in the UK will be diagnosed with prostate cancer. It is the most common cancer in men over the age of 55, and an estimated one in 14 men will develop the condition. A certain type of prostate cancer, known as hereditary prostate cancer, runs in families and can affect men at a much younger age. Prostate cancer occurs when normal, healthy cells, which are regulated in the body, begin to reproduce uncontrollably in the prostate gland. In many cases, growth is small and the cancer can go undetected for many years because it produces few symptoms.

In some cases, prostate cancer grows quickly and may spread to other parts of the body, such as the lymph nodes or bones.

This book covers my personal journey between January 2012 and April 2015, of my fight against this life-shattering disease. As the author, I have gone and come through a horrendous illness and, without a doubt; it has changed my perception of life, people in general and placed my faith firmly in the almighty. During my journey, I have met those suffering far more than I and likened them to heroes and sheroes. Thinking is easy, but acting is difficult, and I found putting my thoughts into actions primarily through words to be the most difficult thing in the world.

If you are reading this book because you or someone dear to you has been diagnosed with some form of cancer, then allow me to empathise with you and hope that this book will help you in some way. I know from my own experiences that, at the time of diagnosis, I refrained from reading anything to do with cancer at all. I suppose my initial attitude was one of 'I'm going to die, so I'll just prepare myself for my own expiry date.' I left it to others, my nearest and dearest, to try to understand what would happen to me and what the future, if any, could hold for me.

I had no interest whatsoever in delving into the minefield of information, misinformation, and facts and figures that could upset or discourage me. Nor was I going to spend loads of money on dubious miracle cures, or alternative medicines. There were so many negative things to think about, I did not ponder for one minute that the possibility I may be that one-in-a-million person to defy the statistics existed. It never crossed my mind until my treatment started to lower my extremely high PSA (prostate-specific-antigen) level, as well as remove and reduce tumours outside my prostate gland.

Only then did I start to believe the impossible and, slowly, my appetite and thirst for knowledge on prostate cancer grew as I began to fight back and revert from my initial mental shutdown. The dawn of seeing things from a positive perspective emerged, as did the opening of my mind to all reasonable possibilities. To read any form of cancer is to discover it is not a competition on who suffers the most; there is no leader board. You have no choice other than to face it head on and get on with life as normal, as much as possible.

'Resilient' was one key word I used to describe myself. However, having a practical sense of just getting on with it and making the best of things best summarised my attitude and approach. At times, the disease gave me false hope; when I thought I was beating it, it roared back with a vengeance. Like a phoenix out of the flames, I rose and fell, only to rise again despite fighting against unimaginable pain. In my opinion, not even any military unit elite could withstand this type of pain during their intense field combat training.

This book may help others at an early stage of their diagnosis or deterring those putting off being checked early like I did from doing so. We men are notorious for ignoring health symptoms and avoiding the doctor's surgery. If we could use sticky tape for all our ailments, we would do so. However, not all medical issues can be fixed so easily; what may be a pesky problem to a man could be a far more serious condition in the making.

In reality, the battle began months, maybe even years before, but my opponent, 'cancer,' had the edge on me. I was only officially alerted to the fight on January 27, 2012. It had been creeping up on me, but I was oblivious. It had given me warning signs, but I ignored them. The frequent need to pee went unnoticed. It took blood in my stool, a niggling back pain and constant nagging from my eldest daughter Celena and partner Grace to convince me to consult with my GP.

I had an MRI scan on January 13, 2012, at St. Mary's Hospital in London. An MRI scan is a Magnetic Resonance Imagining scan, using strong magnetic fields and radio waves to take pictures of the brain or, in my case, the spine. It produces very detailed pictures of the brain and spine. The results were subsequently relayed to my doctor. As I took a pew in the surgery, I noted the disgruntled looks from other patients waiting for their appointments, and could not help but reflect on the roller coaster of events that I had endured over the past few months. My life had been lost in a haze of doctors and hospital visits, and the desperation and frustration were beginning to show in my face. Unawareness of the results only compounded matters further, as I needed answers to my plight, not more excuses or paper exercises.

Late in the summer of 2011, I began to experience progressively worsening back pains. Initially, I experienced the pain only intermittently while jogging. Eventually, however, they worsened until I was unable to exercise or be intimate with my partner without some sort of pain in my lower spine area. In late November 2011, I developed acute radiating pains down my right leg and, barely able to walk, visited my local hospital A&E department. I recall my younger brother Kelly picking me up from home at around 01:30 hours and having to physically lift my right leg to climb into his vehicle, before I could be driven to A&E. He then had to further endure watching me writhe in pain on a hospital trolley for four hours, up to my eyes in paracetamol and codeine. Through this mist of pain, I could see my brother's face contorted with worry and fright over his uselessness to his elder brother's plight. After being medically examined, the doctor suggested that my GP refer me for an MRI scan, as her determination was a possible slipped disc or sciatica.

Up until this point, my body's internal red flashing light had not triggered. For most of my life, I had not been the sickly type of person and rarely visited my GP. However, on this occasion, it was different. I discussed it with my eldest daughter Celena and my partner Grace, both of whom suggested it had to be something else; cancer was never mentioned or a thought. Dangerously, I had failed to give them all the facts at hand, and as such, they were voided of critical information. This was not done intentionally on my part; I never thought the omitted facts would prove so vital.

I decided to adhere to their advice and headed to my GP where, over a six-week period, I was jerked around through surgery practice bureaucracy.

My GP was away on holiday for three weeks and, regardless of the A&E report I submitted to the partner doctor at the surgery, he was reluctant to refer me for the MRI. Instead, he sided with a possible sciatica diagnosis and gave me painkillers, a two-page sheet on back exercises and suggested that I wait for my own GP to return, as I was not an actual patient of his. I was a little disappointed at the remark but I sided with the fact that I was not a patient of this doctor and decided to wait for the return of my own doctor.

Both my partner and daughter were also disappointed but agreed that we wait. Christmas 2011 was upon us, so not much could be done, and as the pain had subsided somewhat, the urgency abated. Once the New Year's festivities were over with, Grace and Celena were on my case again about getting to the doctor and sorting out the MRI scan referral. I attended my surgery and discussed my ailment with my own GP, who had returned from holiday. My GP's advice was to continue with the painkillers and the same back exercise sheet his partner had provided.

The pains came back within days of the New Year, so I returned back to my GP once more. This time, in my mind, I was adamant that I would not leave his office until I was referred for the MRI scan. My GP did not inspire one bit of confidence in me and to say I was pissed would be an understatement. In total, almost four weeks were wasted and valuable medical time lost. After not too much deliberation, a referral letter was agreed upon by my GP for an MRI scan. It was a few weeks between my doctor drafting the referral letter and the actual appointment letter for the MRI scan arriving at my home. I received options for hospitals where the procedure could be provided, and ended up choosing St. Mary's Hospital in London, as this was far more convenient for me.

After I arrived at my appointment, the nurse prepared me for my scan by having me drink what felt like a gallon of water. I was pleased that, as I wore no metal, I did not have to change into a hospital gown, which never seemed to fit me anyway (I wore jogging bottoms and jumper). The nurse then led me into a lovely bright, airy room and introduced me to a smiling radiographer technician, who then informed me about the impending procedure. An MRI is considered as one of the safest medical procedures currently available, and as such, I was not too afraid or worried.

I was supplied with music-playing headphones for the duration of the scan, which lasted approximately thirty minutes. While lying on a flat bed, I was given a panic button to hold onto before the bed moved into the scanner head-first. As I moved through the scanner, a breeze flowed through the tube, which really helped reduce the feeling of claustrophobia. The radiographer operated the MRI scanner, controlling the scanner using a computer positioned in a different room to keep it away from the scanner's magnetic field. I was able to communicate with the radiographer through an intercom. The staff was visually able to see me on a CCTV monitor throughout the scan, and occasionally talked to me during the scan, checking that I was OK.

The scan itself was painless, although, as I lay there, I could hear loud tapping and whirling noises, even through my headphones. These were alarming at times, but, having been warned about the noise prior to entering the scanner, I paid little attention. At times, the tube felt slightly claustrophobic and my mind reflected on my Territorial Army days. One segment of our unit's training involved testing for claustrophobia by entering a maze-like series of underground tunnels as a team of four. Our goal was to make our way through and back out to ground level to a pre-determined point visualised before entering. If you have seen movies of how the Vietcong lived underground during the Vietnam War, you will have some idea of the scenario we faced.

The primary difference between the exercise and my scan was, during those days, I was a fraction of my current weight and size. Coming back to the scan at hand, I suppose the biggest psychological problem for me was lying flat and still for the complete duration of the scan. A support was placed under my legs, but I still suffered pain in my back, buttocks and thighs, which lingered for ages after the scan.

With just two or three inches of space between my body and the machine to spare, I could easily understand how one might panic as those on the outside attempted to identify exactly what was causing my pain. Nevertheless, I was prepared to suffer a little while longer.

Chapter 1 - My Life before Cancer

Born in the late 1950s the eldest of five, I commenced my childhood era during the 1960s and 1970s to an openly exposed world of politics, education, music, TV and fashion. A three political party system existed: Labour, Conservatives and the Liberals. Harold Wilson, Ted Heath and Jeremy Thorpe all hogged the limelight with their government manifests and scandals similar to today's political arena. Education educators were strict, stern and disciplined during my schooling years and bellowing masters maintained discipline or threatened corporal punishment by way of the cane or the lesser of two evils, the slipper. The subject matters taught in no way mirrored today's wider and far more interesting technical subjects. Maybe if these had existed during my youth, I would have veered off into a different profession in life.

The radio produced sounds of the '60s and '70s artists such as Rod Stewart & the Faces, Mick Jagger & the Rolling Stones, Aretha Franklin, Bob Dylan and Otis Redding to mention but a multitude. We listened on our transistorised radios to these stations, some legal, others less so, such as Radio Luxembourg and Carolina where we learned about music and its genres.

Black & White TV sets exposed us further to a multitude of sins of the aforementioned, plus shows such as *This Is Your Life,* hosted by Emanon Andrews, *Ready Steady Go!, Songs of Praise, Opportunity Knocks, Alf Garnett and, of course, The Sweeney*, all of which I remember fondly as they distracted me from school homework.

The era's fashion meant Carnaby Street in central London or King's Road, Chelsea. People from all walks of life flaunted flares and bell-bottoms, miniskirts, tank tops, and platforms (some of which are the rage again, but they do say fashion repeats itself).

The mods, the rockers, the skinheads and the punk rockers were regular features of daily street life and represented the changing face of British society overall. As technology changed, society became more exposed to the woes, ills and politics of the world. As I grew into a young adult and my path, direction and destiny became shaped and moulded for me, I found myself eventually on an unusual doorstep which would encompass a great deal of my past youth.

Some may have called it a highflier lifestyle, others just a professional carrying out his job, but I was the man tasked with watching over the stars, and I don't mean those in the sky. Over a 28-year period, I protected a wealth of entertainment and film stars, as well as corporate entities. I travelled extensively all over the world, primarily in the role of Close Protection Officer, as well as an advance security specialist. Some of the following were my past clients: Bob Dylan, Sade, Seal, Harrison Ford, Patsy Kensit, Rod Stewart, Oasis, Spandau Ballet, Mel & Kim, Bros, Beyonce, Spice Girls, Kelly Rowland, Senior Executives from the French company Matra Space & Defence to mention but a few. Typically working 130 to 140 hours a week without a thought, my 'iron man' mentality prevailed.

The role consumed me; it was my whole life, on the go all the time, physically and mentally. Able-bodied and physically fit, I stood strong and firm in my duties. I actually got into the profession by chance, but have no regrets to be honest. While serving in the British Territorial Army in the 1970s, I met with a number of persons engaged in the entertainment security industry. I was asked if I would be interested in being trained and becoming a Close Protection Officer. It was always a temporary thing and, almost thirty years later, a career unfolded. Along the way, there were issues, which I dealt with discreetly or through my client's legal representatives, or, in some cases, by law enforcement agencies. There was never a dull moment. 'Check, check and check again' was how I operated combined with the cardinal rule of the seven P's: Prior Preparation Planning Prevents Piss

Pot Performance. Alter the Piss Pot to Poor, Poor, if it offends, but it all amounts to the same thing.

My role was to protect these high-profile clients from anything that could cause them harm or embarrassment, from amorous advances, overzealous fans, the notorious paparazzi or, at worst, direct or indirect criminal elements. In addition, I provided what amounted to an A-Z of services, such as intelligence gathering, public relations and personal assistance. I was trained to be totally capable of operating in a multitude of diverse environments, from remote, hostile environments to corporate and executive settings. All of the above presented unique challenges to me, but I never faltered.

As I progressed in the industry and founded my own company, I became the protection officer in-charge of overall security for most assignments. I became known as 'sky man' to those who knew me because I practically lived in the sky. I travelled from one country to another with my clients, using four ten-year passports during my years of service. I must have taken hundreds of flights in this role. My dulcet tone-like voice and refined British accent stood me well in my security briefings, especially with Americans, whose reactions to a black guy with a British accent conversing with them, I found bemusing.

At the beginning, I thoroughly enjoyed and lived for the next assignment, becoming a workaholic. While in the employ of certain clients, I was exposed to the company of other VIPs, celebrities, state and government-level U.S. officials and their own Close Protection teams. Notably, a former U.S. president (at the time a state governor) was one of those I was privy to encounter; rest assured, they enjoyed the music too.

As time rolled on, I began to loathe living out of my suitcase and hotels, as well as the accompanying unhealthy lifestyle apart from my growing family. Other than financially, it was never a rewarding profession. On the contrary, it was mostly thankless, and also, a younger man's profession; the mind and body can only take so much, as father time creeps up on us all in due course. In retrospect, I cringe at all the stupid stuff I did in my earlier young years, apart from the mature well-adjusted adult I have become. If I had my life to live over again and the question 'would this be a field I would enter?' was raised, my answer would be 'probably not.'

Clearly, I had my favourite clients that I enjoyed working with and, on many occasions, I worked with those clients on a regular basis, especially at their request. I developed a close rapport and a professional relationship with my clients and their respective managements, and was renowned for this internationally. It was hard not to develop rapport or close relationships with certain clients, since, at times, I was the only person in close proximity on a regular basis with whom they could rationally discuss issues or vent their frustrations. Nonetheless, discretion and confidentiality were always maintained and never, ever broken.

At the offset, I enjoyed what I did, got satisfaction out of it and, most importantly, I was renowned as a professional. Over the years, I featured in a number of newspapers and international magazine publications, either as a direct feature or a passing mention through clients or other means.

No matter what I did in my life, I was always professional, polite, firm and courteous, and found it kept me in good stead, no matter what I did. Educated to a master's degree level in the study of security management (distance learning), I realised that an opportunity existed in the entertainment industry for risk management services and a somewhat adapted and reduced advance security role.

These fit more into my family lifestyle and career direction. The time came when I had to choose between career and family, and, eventually, I started to provide a specially adapted security role to my clients, forthwith 'Security Advisor' Alfred Samuels was born. By the definition of my particular role, a security advisor is a professional individual who is effective in identifying security requirements for clients and defining reliable and manageable solutions.

This allowed me to offer services in a reduced role, away from the front line of close protection. In a nutshell, the hours were fewer and the physical and mentally demanding aspects reduced to a more comfortable level, though ultimately, I still had to travel internationally, where the money and my focus were at the time. There were times I could not help but think I was being prepared for something out of the ordinary.

Then, along came the diagnosis and cancer struck; in a matter of ten minutes, I received the news that was going to change my life forever and shatter my world around me. My cancer diagnosis shook me up from head to toe and my script on life became very different. To this day, many of my peers still do not know that I have cancer; seemingly, I retired from the circuit after making loads of money and now reside in a hot climate, all of which is so far from the truth.

Advertising my cancer just was not in my makeup. In addition, giving up and saying goodbye to all my dear friends and family was not acceptable in my mind, nor even part of my vocabulary; my struggle had only just begun.

Chapter 2 - The Diagnosis

The date is January 27, 2012, and I am attending my doctor's surgery for the results of an MRI scan. The MRI scan was performed at St. Mary's Hospital, Paddington, London two weeks ago and the results conveyed to my doctor. I recall sitting in the surgery room, waiting for my appointment with my doctor, oblivious to the results of the radiographer report. It was a bright, yet brisk morning and, in myself, I felt quite good physically and mentally, with no real medical conditions about which to complain.

The overhead sign buzzed. "The doctor will see you now," the receptionist told me. I walked to the consultation room, knocked and entered. The room was bright and quiet, and my GP was sitting at his desk. I sat down while he read something from his computer screen. Pleasantries were exchanged and I waited for a conversation.

The conversation commenced with a number of innocent questions thrown at me with regard to the pain I had been suffering. I recall it was if he was looking for a possible alternative answer to my pains, which I could not give him.

Then, like a rapier sword, he thrust the critical statement at me as he turned with his head slightly bowed and eyes failing to meet mine, uttering the words.

"I'm sorry, it's not good news. I'm afraid it's cancer, Mr. Samuels". No one wants to hear the fateful words "you have cancer." The sweat began to bleed through my clothes and the air went still. Neither one of us uttered anything for a moment; it was like that eerie calm before a hurricane swoops in and starts battering your entire house (I experienced one of these in the Caribbean many years ago, something I would not want to ever go through again).

By now, I could see my GP's eyes, which were liquid and showing pain, and I knew how serious he was about the diagnosis. It was clear that he was not the usual type of doctor assiduously rehearsed in the non-brutal technique of telling a patient as gently, but honestly as possible that they have a life-threatening disease by first sizing up their inner resilience, then breaking the sad news.

Stunned, with my head raised to the sky, I exhaled. For a moment, I was in a world of solitude. My GP was talking, but I couldn't hear him, I just saw his lips moving.

Then, it was as if someone un-muted the sound and I came crashing back to reality. 'Why me?' I kept asking myself, aware my GP had just handed me a death sentence.

The scan report demonstrated at least two lesions at the levels L2 and L5, which were entirely consistent with a neoplastic process. There was evidence of vertebral metastases (in layman's terms, that is, it would appear the cancer had spread to my spine), and the radiographer doctor recommended that I be referred to an orthopaedic surgical consultant as a matter of urgency. The whole situation was surreal; 20 minutes prior, I was someone who was a functioning and real part of society, then minutes later, I'm told that I'm no longer going to be a part of that society, and all that I have worked and lived for are to be taken away from me. Flashing through my mind were my thoughts: I'm a father. I've got children. I've got a family counting on me. Why me, why me, why had my life now taken a horrific turn for which I was not ready?

As I re-engaged and started to listen as carefully as my muddled head could manage, I recall my GP saying "We need to get you to the oncology department of your local hospital to have a biopsy carried out which would confirm the diagnosis."

To be honest, I didn't need confirmation; I knew there and then the diagnosis was correct. You see, cancer is in my family history. My mother died in March 1983 of cancer after a seven-year battle, as did her sister six months later, followed by their brother, my uncle about five years later. Over the next fifteen years, two more of my cousins on my mother's side of the family died of cancer, while a number were also diagnosed (still living, including me). I recall my mother's suffering with eye-watering bitterness as she suffered for those seven years before succumbing to breast and lung cancer.

I recall my GP telling me just before I left his consultation room; "If you need to talk about it, just make an appointment at any time" I thought for a moment what a moronic statement. Without a word, I nodded in acknowledgement, got up with paperwork in hand and walked out of the surgery. As I left the surgery, I did not cry; I was too stunned to cry. I have never felt so sad, out of control and helpless as I did at that moment in time. Clearly, I was formally inducted into the world of cancer. My consultation with my GP lasted less than ten minutes; that was all the time I was afforded while being informed about a life-changing disease. An appointment was needed for add-on minutes for further discussion; something was wrong with this scenario, but my mind was totally elsewhere and unable to attempt to try and deal with this.

The walk home was about twenty minutes, but it felt like an eternity; my heart was pounding, pounding, pounding ever so hard now. Fear, pain, alone, confused, apprehensive and dying were just a few of the things floating around in my mind, along with the obvious question of how to tell my family about my condition. There were also the practical aspects to consider. I would need regular treatment and check-ups at a specialist cancer treatment centre and, from the experience of dealing with my mother's cancer care, my condition and the treatment to be undertaken could leave me feeling well below par.

After years of being a father, I was finding it hard to comprehend and accept that it would now be my family's turn to look after me. I walked slowly and aimlessly, but truly felt that something in the form of an angelic being was walking with me. I didn't shed a tear and I recall thinking I wasn't afraid to die, but just wanted to make sure my children were going to be okay. My first instinctive reaction was to collapse into a religious comfort zone and carry on a dialogue with God as to why he had forsaken me when I needed Him most. My mother suffered with cancer for almost seven years and, in that time, she did not once doubt her belief in God.

I personally witnessed and also heard much from her church brethren, so why did I doubt Him now, I asked myself, despite witnessing what he had done for my mother. Right at that moment, I was angry with God for allowing me to get cancer or 'was He indeed punishing me?' was a thought that crossed my mind. At that moment in time, I felt emotionally and physically alone, and, as such, no one could truly know what I was going through in this state of mind. Everyone loses faith at some point in their life. Take me, for example. I grew up in a Christian family and, as a young child, went to church with my mother most Sundays.

I did not have a difficult childhood growing up; I didn't want to go to church, but did not dare to show rebellion. I had no real interest in religion, but my mum and dad's golden rule was "As long as you're in our household, you'll abide by our rules," so Sunday school remained a fixture in my young life.

This lasted until I was 10 years old, before we moved home to an area that did not readily offer Sunday school service. By the time I was seventeen, church was a distant memory, other than on those special occasions, weddings and funerals. Religion was never really rammed down my throat. Spiritual verses were something regularly voiced in our household, and, if I am being honest, some of it stuck with me right into adulthood.

Well, life continued, and it wasn't until my mother became really sick with cancer that I vigorously questioned religion. It was at this point that I started questioning God and His motives.

Why would he allow my dear adorable mother to suffer with cancer for seven years and, subsequently, her family?

After my mother died, I took the question a bit further and asked myself why God would allow suffering to enter into anyone's life. Why had all my prayers not been answered, why so much misery and pain. To believe that prayer could do anything for me, I seriously doubted as I silently screamed for answers.

The years passed, I became an adult and life got more complex and rough, as it does for most. It was at this point that I got really angry at God after losing my home and business during a period of economic downturn. From my point of view, it was as if God didn't care. Fortunately for me, I recalled the times growing up and the spiritual verses that my dad would voice, and these helped my family and I through some lean and turbulent times.

Having gotten through all of that, here I was, once again at the point of losing faith, but a nudge back towards God from my sister was just around the corner. These came in the words of "Sometimes, you have to stop and remember all the things you do have. You've got to be thankful." As is the case with many of us, it was only for a moment that we remain in that doubting frame of mind. This was where my mind rested; holding the thought that, while there is life, there is hope. There would be many more moments of doubt during my illness as my body and mind became weaker and unresponsive, and my mind told me one thing and my body another. It's just human nature.

Chapter 3 The Family The Prognosis

Obviously the focus of attention was now going to be me. I had spent the past thirty years being a tower of strength to everyone around me and never making any demands of them. The next seventy-two hours were to be one of the worst times of my life to date as I went about attempting to inform my children, my partner and my family. Keeping the pain, panic, and sadness from my voice and facial expressions was going to be hard; there was no easy way of doing this other than immediately and coming straight to the point.

I had the classic symptoms of prostate cancer and I had ignored them almost to my peril, in my case the frequent urinal visits to the toilet, the blood in my stool were examples. It took a niggling pain in my lower back and Celena and Grace to constantly prod me before I turned to seek medical advice. I allowed myself time to process the news and get a handle on the diagnosis before I told my children. I suppose I could have hidden the fact that I had cancer for a while and observe how the treatment went but, usually family and close friends learn sooner or later that you have cancer, so that was a non-starter.

As I pondered my thoughts floated on our so called society where the "so called powerful" have mandated that the medical world cut, medicate, eradicate, "chemoate", at peoples bodies. Obviously there is a danger in this acceptance, that this is the best and/or only treatment for cancer. Whatever happened to school of thought on prevention, alternative and complimentary therapies? I wondered, I seriously wondered. However, I was a man of indomitable spirit as they were about to find out.

I decided to rest my mind on my brother Kelly to be the one to spread the news to my siblings, that I had cancer which would assist me a great deal mentally, in lessening the pressure and emotional stress on myself and allow me to concentrate on directly informing my children.

I contacted him by phone and told him that I was coming over to see him that evening. He is my younger brother by five years, who I am very close to and we had enjoyed growing up together. He had looked up to me on many occasions for guidance and help as we grew up, now here I was now looking to him for the same. It's funny how life revolves and reverses. That evening I arrived there about 19:00 hours and thought it would be easy to tell him (in my mind it was all worked out). However, I dithered for a while and paced up and down his dining room area which I know made him nervy before I uttered the following:

"Kelly, Kelly, Kelly," I paused for around five-ten seconds then I said, "I have cancer."

At the time he was at his computer. He immediately looked up with a stunned painful expression, his twisted motionless face showed anguish and immediate loss.

There was a deafening silence for about a further thirty seconds between us before we spoke. I went on to explain in full detail and reverted back to the occasion he had to take me to the hospital in November 2011, whereupon everything became clearer to him.

Having informed him the more difficult task lay ahead, my children. This was not going to be at all easy, not that telling anyone you have cancer ever is. My eldest daughter Celena lived locally, so I called her on her mobile and asked her to pop over to her uncle's home for a chat. Celena's inquisitive detective radar was up and she asked immediately what for. I made some believable excuse and she arrived an hour later.

She came in and sat down next to me across from my brother, we exchanged pleasantries before I attempted to inform her. I recall getting part way before becoming dumbstruck, the words, "I have cancer," never came out of my mouth. They were uttered by my brother as he saw what was happening.

By now, my eyes had welled up and my vision became blurred but my daughter did not cry. I noted that her hands were overactive with a nervous finger twitching. I knew I had to pull myself together and compose myself fast as I had to remain convincing and upbeat and so said so done. Relating the rest came a little more easily, talking about the treatment, and how difficult times were ahead for us as a family, as well as the gradual deterioration of her father's health and possible physical stature.

The day had passed quickly and I realised that my partner had not been informed mostly because she was at work during the day and did not get home until after 19:00 hours. So I had to wait until then before breaking the news. For me my regret was not being able to be next to her and hold her hand and tell her face to face.
This may have lessened the impact but cancer is cancer and there is never an easy way to tell anyone that you have the disease. I recall the moment as a nineteen year old young man when myself and my siblings were gathered at home and my father and mother gave us the news that our mother had breast cancer. Shocked, visibly shaken were just a few of our emotions but nobody cried until the day she died.

At the appointed time I picked up the telephone and made the call. She answered with her gleeful but weary self and we exchanged pleasantries, then I told her the sad news. The eeriness turned into tears, the tears turned into garbled words only some of which I caught "Oh no, no, no, no, Al No" the remainder of our conversation was had with her in tears. I had told the person who I loved and was intimately involved with that I was possibly going to die and no longer a part of her life. It hurt; it really hurt me emotionally when I uttered those words. I recall Grace did not go to work the following day as she was far too upset to face it. I knew that we both needed time to digest the news and then decide on the course of action and subsequently the treatment.

With this done my other daughters and sons needed to be informed which again was no easy task. My son Nathan and daughter Kira lived in Birmingham. My other son James and daughters Sam and Lajade all lived in different parts of London.

I decided to deal with everyone separately except, my two children in Birmingham who I decide I would telephone jointly. Before calling them I called their mother, informed her first, and got her to arrange that they both be available to take my call. I clearly recall that conversation, with the phone on loudspeaker; I conveyed the sad and distressing news to them. There was again that deafening silence from them both before their tear jerking voices came across "Oh dad, oh dad so sorry."

I assured them as best as a father could that I was going to fight this disease, under no circumstances were they to believe that my battle with cancer had been lost, and that I would keep them informed and in the loop as to treatment and progress. One would have thought that after each revelation it would become easier, I can tell you that it was far from that as the emotional dagger twisted deeper each time in relating the information.

My daughter Lajade was next in line and I decided to go to her mother's home (though once again I called her mother first before arriving and informed her of the situation). Upon arrival, I went into the living room and sat down with her mother first as our daughter was upstairs.

We exchanged a few words whereupon her mother beckoned our daughter downstairs. Lajade was aged eighteen at the time.

She came into the front room with her usual bouncy smiling full-of-life self, but I knew this imminently was about to change. We hugged and exchanged pleasantries, and I sat down. My daughter sat across the way from me and looked at me inquisitively and said "Daddy, what's wrong?" as she sensed something was not right. Once again the bearer of sad news had to carry out an unpleasant duty as I decided not to sugar-coat anything. I uttered the destructive and devastating words *Daddy has cancer*. My daughter jumped up out of her chair as I observed the fright and hurt in her eyes. The tears rolling down her cheek (you know something even as I write now my eyes are filled with tears and that blurry unfocused vision exists) and came over to where I was seated and sat beside me and rested her head on my right shoulder and cried further. I can tell you now children will bring to their knees the biggest, baddest and hardest man when they cry for you.

For a few minutes we hugged before I departed from her home again. I left her with my thoughts that I had every intention of battling the cancer and it was just another battle I intended to win. She insisted she wanted to walk me to my car and she did. My son James came to see me at home with his godfather a week later whereupon I informed them both. Once again the look of loss was upon his face as he gathered his thoughts. James just said "Dad, we just got to spend as much quality time together then." My other daughters Amber and Jenelle who resided overseas, were contacted by phone and given the sad news, both were upset at the news and responded tearfully. Distraught, lonely, tearful along with negative thoughts were just a few words and feelings which started to become familiar within me. I suppose in hindsight it was all a little rushed as I was not able to give them all the medical facts.

I did feel that to overwhelm them with too much information could cause them to have a hard time processing all; after all for me it was the first in a series of conversations that we were to have. I gave them the information I had and did not lie. Children have a way to sense when something is wrong and you are not telling the truth and that was not the relationship that existed between me and my children. I knew that it would take a couple of days for those who loved me, to process it all before the avalanche of questions would be forthcoming and making myself ready for that was to be my next task at hand. Three days later I was sitting in the waiting room of the oncology department at my local hospital where I was seen by a consultant oncologist. The last seven days had really been mentally and physically taxing on me. I was beginning to look pale, tired and old more-so after informing my partner and children of my life-limiting disease. I felt at a loss but knew optimism was the foundation of courage. I needed to exemplify this more so to my children than others, as I also needed to show them that I would not be that predictable cancer patient. Even in illness a parent has to demonstrate and make sure their children have the necessary tools that they need to deal with any form of life-limiting disease and the challenges ahead, should this befall them.

Bloods were taken from my arm as well as a biopsy carried out.

I returned to the hospital a week later, for consultation with my oncologist and the results were laid before me. My PSA was recorded as over 507ng/ml (normal is considered to be below 3.5ng/ml for someone of my age at the time). My Gleeson score was registered at seven and my biopsy results were confirmed as positive for metastatic prostate cancer with a staging level of four recorded. The diagnosis had come back and it was now officially clear that I certainly had advanced metastatic prostate cancer, arising from the prostate gland originally.

My oncologist discussed in-depth with me the way forward and a clinical treatment course was offered to me. This was to be the randomised controlled 'Stampede' drugs trial programme, which is a multi-arm drug trials looking at various treatment options for patients with high risk, locally, advanced or metastatic prostate cancer. The medical definition of "STAMPEDE" is Systemic Therapy in Advancing or Metastatic Prostate Cancer – Evaluation of Drug Efficacy. Clinical research trials are carried out to answer questions about investigational medicines. This involves several phases of

Clinical research to see if they are safe and effective before doctors prescribe them.

Strangely though the process for selection was carried out by a computer with information inputted by medical professionals. As previously stated this was a multi-arm randomised controlled drug trial. The newer drugs in this trial were Zoledronic Acid (Zometa), Docextaxel (Taxotere) and Abiraterone (Zytiga). These aimed to make a fair comparison between new treatments and the existing treatment to see which works the best. A controlled trial compares two or more groups of people: a research group who receive the research treatment and a control group who receive the standard treatment. This allows researchers to see whether the treatment they are testing is any more or less effective than the existing treatment.

Now you reading this are probably as confused as I was at the time, much of this information flew straight over my head as I clearly was not a medical professional. I just wanted the layman's terms put to me to enable me to understand properly. Admittedly, at the time this new advance treatment for advanced prostate cancer was viewed and hailed as an extended life saver. Back in the late 1980s and 1990s the projected survival time for a man diagnosed with evident metastatic prostate cancer was about eighteen to thirty-six months. For me personally going through cancer was a journey I did not want to make but I had to. Once again, I had to travel a cancer journey but this time I was on the receiving end; I was the patient. Here I was facing the second most frequently diagnosed cancer globally.

I knew it was going to take a lot of travelling for me to get back on the road to good health. Knowing if I did not pick the right road my life could be in danger.

Fortunately consultation with my partner who was on hand and who herself was a medical professional, but not a cancer specialist aided me in understanding and making a formative decision. I could not but think if I did not have such a partner how would I have coped and I questioned how other people in similar situations coped also. Let me not forget my children were also playing their part by carrying out their own independent research. After much family deliberation, it was agreed that I should join the Stampede trial programme. The option to remove my prostate had long passed as the cancer had spread outside the prostate gland and I was now in deadly trouble.

Here I was this active virile British born Afro-Caribbean male whose life had now taken an absolute 180 degree turn around. The core of my masculine identity was now affected and mentally this was to become extremely difficult for me to deal with. However in the grander scheme of things, I was alive and that was far more important. My treatment was to be different and the traditional path was not to be taken. Instead chemotherapy tablets along with a hormone injection administered every three months was the path I would undertake. I decided to keep a daily personal and symptom diary between March 2012 and April 2015, of which personal and intimate information from this diary of my treatment, side effects, psychological mind set, fatigue to skin irritation to fevers and chills and physical demeanour were recorded.

At the time I really don't know what made me keep a dairy. The weary process of going through the daily chore of unscrewing the cap of a pen in my hand and jotting down in my notebook everything that happened and everything that would be felt for the foreseeable future, including the surprises just did not sit well with me. By placing my words on paper it inadvertently aided me in understanding some of what was going on with me medically and also took some of the pressure off my mind. Being part of the pioneering process in a cancer drugs trials programme meant a great deal. In most cancer drug trials it can be up to eight years before a particular drug is actually approved and made available to the public. The question I asked myself was, did I have eight years to wait?

Nonetheless, I was a part of history; imagine if this was the complete cure and absolute answer to the cessation of prostate cancer deaths. I could not imagine anything more rewarding than being a part of history, and if it did not work out at least I would have gained a few more years to my life.

Chapter 4 - SYMPTOM DAILY DIARY 2012

This diary was written on the basis of maybe its contents could add something new to the cancer table. It should not be taken that the cliché of writing a cancer diary is going to compound the impossibility of writing in it anything other than what has already been written, over and over; same story, same ending.

29 March 2012,

Today being my earth day (My Birthday) I attended my local hospital, for an appointment with my consultant oncologist to discuss the treatment that I will undergo. The treatment recommended was as a result of a computer being fed personal information about me and my illness and then throwing out which arm of the Stampede treatment programme I should undergo (clearly we have reached the age of machines replacing good old fashion doctors it seems). I drew arm G of the stampede trials programme "hormone treatment and abiraterone" - Whilst in treatment group G, I will receive a Prostap hormone injection plus a course of abiraterone tablets. The hormone treatment is standard for patients with advanced metastatic prostate cancer. The Hormone therapy is intended to reduce the testosterone levels in my body and will be administered chemically, by an injection.

This will be administered once a month for the first six months and then once every three months thereafter.

The abiraterone tablets will be taken as a daily dose of 1g (four tablets) for up to two years. The tablets are to be taken on an empty stomach. In addition, I will need to take Prednisolone (which are steroid tablets) daily whilst I am on the abiraterone tablets. Elated is just a small way to describe how I feel today, not because it's my birthday. Something which I had actually ceased celebrating, due to my mother dying of cancer on the 25th of March 1983 which, was five days short of my birthday. The oncology hospital staff all seemed genuinely happy about me drawing Arm G of this trial programme also and that felt encouraging.

I am amazed at the amount of people that I see during my treatment visits who are involved in my care it is most definitely a team effort. I also received in hand the second Hormone Prostap injection from the Cancer ward which I have to take to my GP and have administered by the surgery nurse. Sounds back to front to me, I haven't got my head around that process as yet. My oncologist discussed in detail with me the daily medication treatment that I needed to take to treat the disease and obviously stay alive.
These came in the form of tablets and were as follows:-

Abiraterone acetate tablets 250mg – Four tablets once daily on an empty stomach. No food to be consumed for at least two hours before the dose and for at least one hour after the dose.

Omeprazole Gastro-resistant capsules 20mg – One to be taken twice a day. These two drugs were to be taken together each morning. Prednisolone tablets 5mg. - One tablet once a day with or just after food or a meal Morphine Sulphate controlled release tablets 10mg – Two to be taken twice a day Avoid alcohol – If sleepy do not drive/use machines

Ibuprofen Tablets 400mg – One to be taken three times daily with or just after food or a meal.

Oramorph Oral Solution 10mg/5ml Morphine sulphate – Which was to be used only in case of breakthrough pain ONLY. In other words to be taken when the pain was severe between regular medication times.

This was to be my life and already I was dreading it, what a way to exist I thought but, the show must go on. It is a show in my mind playing my part on the stage of life and its revolving dramas before me.

30 March 2012

Today my arm felt a little sore from the prostap injection, which will now be administered as part of the treatment programme. I felt somewhat weepy, which apparently is one of the known side effects that I had been warned about. For no reason at times during the day, I have just wanted to cry. My eyes well up and my inner emotions just seem to play total havoc even if I am watching a sad movie or an advert for example famine relief showing undernourished and needy children. But I say to myself put a soldiers face on and brave it Alfred. I think to myself, I know this is a hard road that I am about to travel, but my children, my partner and some close and dear friends are there supporting me through this and my thoughts regularly fall on them.

This support is without a doubt helping me. I attended an appointment at my doctor's surgery with my brother as part of the follow up process. A thought entered my mind as we sat with the doctor and discussed matters which I felt obliged to ask. It was the inevitable question 'how long?' How long did I have to live was the question, of course, I understood that it would be unreasonable of me to expect him to know, with any certainty, when I'm likely to die if I have the treatment. I'm sure it's different for everyone, and his answer would only be based on statistics, but perhaps he would give me a general idea: years… months… weeks?

As he answered he uttered, *"Do not make any long term plans."* I looked at my brother who had sat silently throughout the consultation and saw his face twitch uncomfortably, but still he remained silent.

In between, my brain had taken a little while to fully comprehend the reply as I focused on the clock on the wall time's increment decline, and then I arrived at his words –*'do not make any long term plans'*. Suddenly it struck me, with all the force in the fullest sense of the statement that a cricket player hit the ball for six, that this could actually be his answer. I was mortified and shocked, (not what I was expecting from this appointment) before I'd had properly started out on the treatment road the spectre of death was hovering before me. It was a culturally familiar diagnostic term and I had to come to terms with as well as a difficult real-life calculation, jokingly I wondered if our TV remote battery would run out first or not.

My body's cells were not in agreeance and were over reacting as I attempted to adjust and maintain a reasonable calmness to my exterior, more so in the presence of my brother. It was quite hard to rapidly absorb the notion that someone though a doctor was forecasting my demise, my head began to hurt as the weariness of it all started to set in. I felt like just nodding a thank you and take my leave of the surgery and its pessimism, regardless of the felt brevity of the statement, everyday life still remained before me, though shortened. I could do one of two things: sit in sadistic silence, do nothing at all, and give up, or make up my mind to fight under the guise of a glimmer of hope and optimism that existed for a selected few, "God's chosen ones." With that said, I decided to take a long-term view and get on with what was ahead. Without further ado, we left the surgery with not much else being said between my brother and me. I think for us it had all been said already.

31 March 2012

Woke up today in some discomfort, lower back area L2, L3 are feeling very warm and in myself I feel unwell. Can't place my finger on exactly what's wrong other than I don't feel myself at all. My children are taking me out tonight for a meal, can't let them down or let them see that I don't feel up to it, they are my inspiration to fight this disease and seeing them more regular really helps though I am attempting to hide from them the moments of weepiness that seem to be overcoming me now. I suspect it will be more than my children at my meal tonight

(I wasn't born yesterday smile).

Well, as I suspected it was a surprise birthday meal at the Mango Rooms (Thai Food) Buckingham Palace Road London, opposite Buckingham Palace itself). Excellent evening raised my spirits no end and desire and will to live.

To say I felt special was an understatement, surrounding me were my some of my close family and friends it felt good to be alive today. My dear brother Kelly and daughters Celena and Lajade were the chief instigators in making this surprise party happen. My daughters looked like polished diamonds and there and then I realised how much they had grown up.

I felt very tired after the evening's entertainment and my lower back area was still very warm. I have made a physical note to let my consultant know what's going on at my next appointment. On reflection the evening was overshadowed by my eldest daughter Celena informing me that my other daughter Kira, who resides in the Midlands, had called her that evening crying, in fact bawling' she had rung her big sister to let her know that my condition had really hit her and she felt I had changed as a person. All I could say was my love for her and all my children was intact.

My emotions were clearly all over the place, yes I cried as my eldest related to me as I know it affected her also. There and then I realised I needed to be stronger, but, how could I when the side effects are affecting me so much. I feel that I am losing control of me as a person and I need me to be a part of the fight process. God, what am I going to do, please show me what to do please.

1 April 2012

Woke today feeling exhausted primarily from the hip down and my hands felt drained, virtually stayed in bed all day. May have pulled a right calf muscle as I have pain in that area also. Mentally, I feel okay other than wondering why I am so exhausted; will talk with oncologist tomorrow as I have an appointment. What strikes me is how fast I seemed to have been physically incapacitated. Funnily enough, I still have this spiritual feeling of someone or something is walking beside me each day as I go through this illness. From the day I received my diagnosis from my doctor I have felt this way that "I am not alone in my struggle".

2 April 2012

I awoke today feeling a little discomfort in my lower back area, no pain, just discomfort. I have an appointment at the hospital today at 15.35 hours. Met with oncology doctor and signed consent document for Stampede trials programme admission. Informed doctor about pain in back area, whereupon he examined my lower back, but found nothing that overly concerned him, however he stated that it could be a side effect of the prostap injection. Prescription given to me for steroid tablets which are to be taken along with taking the abiraterone tablets. The hospital Stampede trials nurse for the trial programme discussed the whole process with me again. I then attended the hospital ward, to obtain my first batch of abiraterone tablets. Felt very uncomfortable at this location as this was an actual cancer ward and advance cancer patients were visible and audible to me.

To make matters worse a day after April fool's day. I was made to wait for two-and-a-half hours in the waiting room only to be forgotten by staff who had locked up and gone home for the day. You hear of these things but never think for one moment that you will experience such a moment but I did today. I made the staff on the ward aware of what had happened, they looked stunned as I related. They attempted to access the room where the drugs were held, but could not find the keys to do so, so no drugs were obtained. Furious was not the word, I felt like a prize dick, but more to the point I felt totally alone, forgotten and given up on already, and we had not even started my treatment. Was this the pattern to come I asked myself?

How could they do this? My two-and-a-half hours wait subjected me to listening to other cancer patients discussing their issues at a time and state that I really did not care to hear it. I felt like signing off the programme there and then, but common sense prevailed as up until this point all medical attention had been professional and humane. Nonetheless a complaint was going to be registered. It made me feel like I was a nobody - nothing! How dare they do that? My thoughts revolved around getting sleep as they say "sleep on it" before making possible irrational actions or otherwise. I came home and decided to have an early night. Night, Night, a thought for tomorrow came to mind "Worrying does not empty tomorrow of its troubles... It empties today of its strength.

3 April 2012

Well, another day and the good lord has allowed me to awake to which I am eternally grateful. Feel a little tired from the thighs down and lower back area. Having slept fairly well, I am now ready to tackle the incident of yesterday at my local hospital.

I immediately wrote an email to the hospital Stampede trials nurse, who is the research nurse appointed to the programme and my point of contact. Having sent the email I felt better in myself. I waited for a few hours before I followed this up with a telephone call to ensure the email had been received.

At around 09:15 hours I received an apology via the phone though somewhat "Denialish" but only to be expected typical corporate shit. I was required to attend the hospital at 10.00 hours today to receive my unissued abiraterone & steroid medication tablets. Upon my arrival everything was packed and waiting for me... and so it bloody well should be.

The whole process from arrival to departure took 12 minutes. All this upheaval and stress for 12 minutes after a two-and-a-half hours wait yesterday.

How do you equate this? My oncologist, has offered to open a clinical incident form to further investigate matters. Let's see where it goes, personally speaking I am of the opinion I just wasted valuable air and effort! Hmmmmm.

Met up with another of my daughters 'Samantha' today to inform her of my condition as she remains unaware that I have cancer. Felt choked, but glad I did it, especially as she took it fairly well. Feeling very tired in my body and mind (these are becoming daily events) need to get home and sleep. Arrived home at 14.25 hours. Going to get some sleep now write more when I get up.

It's 19.35 hours and I am awake now felt physically weak but rested. My thought process seems to be pointing me in the direction of getting stronger emotionally - Recalled my own mother's fight with cancer and her faith which kept her going throughout her seven year illness.

I have got to stay strong; I have got to get stronger are regular sentiments I say to myself. Just looked back at a text sent to my eldest daughter Celena yesterday evening "Woke up still feeling totally livid and until put pen to paper and vocally voice my discontent it will continue to consume me...I am totally outraged and thank god it was not a medical procedure that went wrong though in a way it is... Denial of medication is what it amounts to."

Well, I certainly did do that this morning. "Don't let it get to you Alfred. You have much more ahead and will need your strength," is what I said to myself (enough said). My thigh area in both legs are feeling tender.

My neck is slightly painful and tender along with a few pains on the left side of my chest rib cage area. However, the feeling as if I had pulled a muscle in my calf is no longer an issue and seems to have worked itself out.

4 April 2012

Officially commenced the Stampede trials programme today. Abiraterone tablets taken today at 08:30 hours as directed. One hour later additional tablets taken.

16:45 hours no side-effects as yet, just stiff back in L2, L3 areas of lower back, but in general throughout the day felt well.

23:45 hours took morphine 10mg tablets along with other tablets. Lower back area still playing me up, but still feel good. Getting an early night, not much more to say. Maybe tomorrow I'll have more to say. Lord thanks for being with me today some days I forget to say a simple thank you to you but I know you understand.

5 April 2012

I awoke this morning with a hell of a neck ache on the left side not sure what that's about. 09:00 hours abiraterone tablets as prescribed and directed. One hour later additional tablets taken. My back still playing me up, but other than that I feel good. Heard from my daughter Kira via text she is trying to get to grips with it, she says "Hi, I'm sorry for the late reply just got credit on my phone I didn't want to bother you with how I feel I just need time and I'm just finding it really hard however, I'm here for you 1000% and positive thinking equals positive outcomes.... Love You xxx".

Well, what can I say other than a lump came into my throat and a little tear, she is very perceptive, more than she knows or realises love her so much, at times we are at a distance, but we love each other dearly it's a strange situation at times but what's most important is the reciprocal love that exists from all of my kids. As the evening draws on my back is playing me up and is becoming more painful feels like I am back peddling. Lower and upper back areas are painful. I also notice I am feeling very tired along with a slight swelling under my left eye. My current mood is that of slightly weepish and unwell. Grace came over and picked me up from home for the Easter weekend.

6 April 2012

03:30 hours woke up feeling intermittent pain in the left forearm of my right arm, My chest is all tingling and painful. Experiencing hot flushes also, my head is spinning what's happening to my life, to my family's life also. Shooting pains down the right foot, which make me wince somewhat. Attempted to go to the toilet stood up and right foot is all very painful could hardly place body weight on foot to walk to the bathroom. Most of the pain is in the area of the right toe and pad of toe area. Pain and discomfort lasted until 04:05 hours.

Throughout the night foot remained tender. No problem or discomfort when passing urine. Right eye is still puffy under the eye. Incorrectly stated yesterday, which eye was puffy for clarification, it is the right eye. Woke up again at 09:10 hours and took tablets as directed. One hour later additional tablets taken. Still having problems with right foot pain in right toe and pad of foot, no swelling of toe or foot though.

Managed to walk to the toilet, but something is not right, will monitor (I have telephone contact numbers of hospital should I need to call).

Having woken up properly now and opened the curtains it is noted that my left side rib cage area is showing signs of inflammation, the skin surface is red and has spread over an area measuring (2" x 2"). This is the second and third rib area. Grace has been such a comfort and excellent friend and carer, sometimes when she talks to me, I respond in a rough manner, it's not meant and I realise after, so just to say Grace sorry for any offence but it's not the real me as you know, without you half of me would not manage and I wonder at times how long I would and could go on for.

16:20 hours attempted to walk and found a reoccurrence of this morning's pain, right foot instep pad very painful, after 20 minutes pain moved to heel area and a painful spot was very apparent. Ankle felt numb which lasted for about 25 minutes, after which I was able to walk again without pain. Today being Good Friday dinner was great and then I spoilt it, whilst around the dining table I became very emotional and I broke down in tears. I have no real idea why I just did. I came over all emotional and had to excuse myself from the table, these are the moments when I feel vulnerable and weak.

My right foot is still smarting, but I am able to walk on it, but something is not right about it. I'll give it another 24 hours and if no improvement I will contact the oncology department out of hours telephone number that I was given. I looked out into the garden this evening and the flowers were daffodils blooming along with dead shrubs, could only think of me buried there and "pushing up the daisies and daffodils" expression came to my mind. Had a game of Scrabble with Grace ended the evening... I won... smile.

7 April 2012

I awoke at 06:10 hours still have a pain in my left foot, however, not as bad as yesterday. 09:05 hours abiraterone tablets taken as a directed. 10:20 hours additional tablets were taken as directed. In myself, I feel generally well just a few pains in various parts of the body but dull in intensity.

My thoughts lie in have I, have we made the right decision as regards the stampede trial as these aches and pains continue and it's me feeling the intensity.14:50 hours my foot is not hurting as much though a slight pain is apparent, but unlike yesterday have decided to hold off on contacting hospital and will keep an eye on it for a few more days.

A realisation hit me today in that this week has been a hell of a week and has tested my physical and mental strengths unlike at any time before in my life. Spiritually, I have become closer to an invisible entity as such, as well as myself if that makes sense.

Yes, I have advanced prostate cancer at my current age of 54. Though, 11 years prior to November 2001 I should have died without a doubt. I crashed the car I was driving whilst in the Caribbean island of Jamaica at 90 mph in the rain and on a bend and the question asked now and then was, "how did I survive that?"

Well, only God knows why he sent those angels to protect me and once again that feeling exists now. I'm going to pull through this because God has a greater plan for me that lays ahead. I find things that I was unable to physically do a few months ago I am gradually able to do now with more ease. I sit here looking at the TV, but find myself regularly reflecting on my life bisecting and dissecting as much of it as I can remember. Why me to get cancer? Why me?

8 April, 2012

Easter Sunday and another day I'm allowed to wake up to and be a part of this world. Right foot not so painful this morning. 09:10 hours abiraterone tablets taken as prescribed.

10:40 hours additional tablets taken slightly later than usual. Contacted my local hospital and spoke with oncology doctor on duty. Discussed problem with Dr. she suggested it could be gout, but suggested as the pain was gradually decreasing each day that I should wait until Tuesday and contact the research nurse and pass on symptoms for their attention. Personally speaking I can't see it being gout.

Decided I would cook today at Grace's home. Felt real good that I prepared a meal for her and her son Josh. Even more so that they enjoyed it. I did put an awful amount into it and it meant a lot for their kind comments. Felt exhausted afterwards though, especially having stood on my feet for a number of hours. Had been warned to stay cool at all times if possible. Another side effect of the hormone injection was hot flushes so cooking was becoming a thing of the past it seemed.

Need to address this problem as this could become an issue in the long term. Spent Saturday with Grace and we had a good talk about my past, in particular an event that suggested I should be dead. In September 2001, whilst holidaying in the Caribbean I was involved in a head-on car collision, it was stupid, senseless, painful and carnage. As she said, I truly had an angel beside me that day. We discussed some of the countries that I had travelled throughout the world and things I had seen and how they affected my overall perspective on life. Our talk was deep and meaningful and I realised then how much I cared about her. I did wonder though if she would be better off in life with someone else, who could make her far happier than I could now and oh how she deserved it.

At this moment in time due to the varying side effects of the drugs I cannot be as intimate towards her as I had previously. In our intimate conversations, she had indicated to me she was not worried and wanted our relationship to carry on regardless. I cannot but wonder what she really thinks at times as I am sure she keeps much to herself in those "Secret Places" we have. Easter passed quickly and tomorrow I travel back to my home. Our time spent is all but over too quick to be honest. I looked at the reflexology foot diagrams and realised how spot-on the areas that I am having pains in relate to my condition. Children have not contacted me today, made me feel very sad. I look forward to hearing from them as they are what I live for. Felt extremely tired as I wrote my notes, most definitely an early night. 22:34 hours last of daily tablets taken.

9 April 2012

02:30 hours, woke with shooting pains in my left foot which kept me awake. I also have a feeling something is not right. I texted two of my daughters who had gone out night clubbing together to see if all was well. At 04:10 hours they responded with "they were fine". Must be something else going on just don't know what yet, I just felt apprehensive about something. Took some digital pictures of myself today, personally speaking my facial features look drawn and tired in most of them and in my face I can see how ill I am, it never used to be like that. Maybe it's because I'm getting older, I'll use that reason for now as it makes me feel better emotionally. Realised that I did not make a note of tablets taken as prescribed at 09:05 hours; 10:10 hours respectively. At 23.00 hours last of my daily tablets were taken.

10 April 2012

09:15 hours, abiraterone tablets taken as a prescribed. Felt fairly well today, no pain in either foot to complain about. Contacted my doctor at the surgery to request a repeat prescription of morphine MST. The receptionist could not find repeat requests on computer referred matter to my doctor. This surgery is getting on my nerves; I'm physically going there to sort this out. Contacted local hospital spoke with research nurse who had apparently spoken with on-the-call oncologist doctor about pain in my foot. The matter is to be referred to the oncologist with a possibility of attending hospital prior to my April 18 appointment. Waiting for confirmation of the date and time.

Contacted Macmillan nurses and discussed financial assistance, referred to a benefits job centre to seek disability allowances. Additional information to be mailed to me for other benefits, felt real sad about going this route, not used to this at all. Attended doctor's surgery picked up my prescription at 17:20 hours 120 tablets two packs of 60. Absolutely tired when I got in at 23:10 hours, my back was also playing me up, as I had misjudged a step today when getting off the bus and slightly jarred my back.

Very tiring and stressful day only complicated by the incompetent doctor's surgery receptionist, fortunately I had recorded telephone conversation via Skype with an MP3 recording of the conversation that I had earlier with her which totally showed her incompetence.

My personal finances are causing me great concern as I have exhausted personal saving funds and business funds. I am waiting for an outstanding amount owed to my company which would keep me and the company afloat for many more months whilst other contracts that I am about to be awarded comes to fruition in the next few months from a foreign government client. I am of the opinion that cancer is certainly not biased, it strips you of everything, including finances and if you think sympathetic ears are listening then think again.

Cancer does not define me, but how I live and fight with cancer does define me. Back pain increasing. I am wondering if I should increase dosage of morphine again, will contact doctor to seek further advice. 23:30 hours last of daily medication taken.

11 April 2012

I awoke at 02:30 hours with a very warm feeling which was felt in the right-side of my stomach, just below my right breast. No pain was felt, but the bodily area of contention, was much warmer than any other area of my stomach. At 09:04 hours abiraterone tablets taken as prescribed. One hour later additional tablets were taken as per instructions. Contacted Macmillan nurses.

I had a relaxing day today and decided to watch a DVD that my brother Kelly had bought for me from the United States entitled *Forks over Knives*. I have to say this book may have helped further to save my life, the documentary DVD revolves around all foods and plant diet and states that diet is so much more important than anyone thought before.

Sickness is caused by the food we eat and quality of life is within reach. (Ancient Egyptian proverb) "One quarter of what you eat keeps you alive the other three quarters keeps your doctor alive". The DVD states that diet can reverse cancer type's breast/prostate. Further, it adds that there are people who have had a metastatic prostate cancer all over their body and who have gone through spontaneous remission and being cured. You are in control of your life. If a lady of over seventy years can state the following, "if I had a healthy body and was putting the right food in it I can beat this cancer," and she did.

The DVD gave me a lot of hope that as we age, we can beat the degenerative diseases that people get. As mentioned by participants "eat to live and don't live to eat".

Makes a whole heap of sense to me, food for thought, excuse the pun though, smile.

12 April 2012

09:00 hours abiraterone tablets taken as prescribed. One hour later additional tablets taken. Received telephone call from the hospital Stampede trials nurse who was just checking on how I was with regards to the foot pains that I had been complaining about. Today I found myself reflecting on my condition again and the lead up to the diagnosis. On October 2011 at around 01.00 hours my brother Kelly took me to the A&E unit at my local hospital, the next two-and-a-half hours he watched me writhe in pain unlike anything I had ever endured.

The look on his face I will never forget as I shook the hospital trolley that I lay on. No matter what drugs they gave me the pain would not subside, it was awful and he could do nothing to help me. It hurt me emotionally to know what he went through as I lay there writhing in pain. Even now as I write a tear rolls down my face. Watching a loved one in so much pain is something not to have happen. Little did we know that it was cancer that I was suffering from. Six months later the pain is a distant memory, but the illness is not. The financial strain is now becoming a problem for me and keeping my business affairs afloat is a daily burden and stressful.

These head pains I suffer with, I can only attribute to the stress I'm undergoing. How can I get through this? Lord only knows that I am trying. Even the simplest of tasks I find extremely hard, such as bending down and tying my shoes, putting my clothes on are all making me breathless. 20:00 hours felt pain in my upper back area again; especially when I arched my back I would get a dull pain. The pain is just below my right shoulder blade. This is not the first time I have had this pain and like certain other pains it comes and goes. In general, though, I feel good within myself compared to a few weeks ago. I can only say a feeling of general wellness exists. 23:00 hours tablets taken as prescribed.

13 April 2012

08:50 am tablets taken as prescribed. 09:50 am additional tablets taken. Spent a few hours in the park today, really felt good to be alive and around nature, along with my partner Grace, who was on a day off from work. We took some great pictures which made me feel good about myself.

Today I realised that these special moments that we share make the difference. The pain started again in the area below the shoulder in my upper back; also my right leg and foot were painful. For the first time I have seen how my illness has affected Grace, a few times I winced in pain and she caught sight of this, I noticed that she disappeared from the lounge for a while. Upon her return I noted the redness in her eyes and tissues in her pocket.

I decided to have a heart to heart talk with her and asked her why she had been crying. She responded by saying, "I just don't know what to do when I see you in so much pain, I feel helpless." I asked her whether she talks to anybody about what is going on with me. There was no answer so I figured she was all alone in her world. Felt very tearful and felt as if it was me that made her feel this way. She went on to say that there had been other occasions whilst I was away that she had been tearful and despondent.

I recall telling her a story from my past. 20 years ago I had visited this spiritualist in Luton where he told me then that I would have one serious illness in my life.

Well, it's here now in my face and I have to deal with it, not try to deal with it. I really am glad that I'm not around the children to let them see the pain that I go through at times, as this would shake me up inside and them also. Well, it's almost midnight and I have been up from 07:20 hours in fact earlier. The good thing is that I don't feel as tired as I had been in the past, usually I would have had an afternoon nap by now. Last set of daily tablets taken at 23.58 hours.

14 April 2012

09:00 hours tablets as per instructions. 10:00 hours additional tablets taken with breakfast. Felt slightly uneasy in body, but physically okay. Eldest daughter Celena called and we had a heart-to-heart conversation as regards family and medical history. Quite a long conversation was had whereupon, I realised I needed to inform my children about more information as relates the family medical history. I was surprised that certain members of my family were very affected by my condition and how it also reminded them of our late mother.

15 April 2012

09:15 hours tablets taken as prescribed. 10:30 hours additional tablets taken. Noticed blood stains in my underwear two spots in the penis area. No idea that this was there though this must have happened on

Friday as my underwear was changed then. I've not noticed any blood when I urinate in the toilet.

Put a real dampener on my day worrying to say the least.

An afterthought the discharge must have occurred whilst I was wearing my underwear as do not wear underwear to bed and there are no signs of blood in the bed. Between 12:40 and 14:00 hours fell asleep as I was not feeling too well. Awoke feeling okay, no real pain as such. Throat is just feeling slightly sore used TCP to gargle a few times throughout the day. It's funny when you watch TV and see cancer ads how you dismiss them.

Now when an advert comes on and I am so affected by it to the point of blocking it out of my mind. A particular advert that gets me every time is the Macmillan nurses advert where a female interviewed says, "When I was told I had cancer I could not believe I had cancer".

16 April 2012

09:10 hours tablets taken as per instructions. 10:00 hours additional tablets taken. Slight nasal congestion coming on over the last few days. Calf muscle still tender at times (right leg). Feeling stressed over business matters, as I know my finances are in a dire state. Received Macmillan forms not sure if I qualify, need to discuss with them further. My lower back feeling painful, maybe I overdid some room adjustments causing extra stress on my back. I sat and stared out of my window today at the pouring rain. Listening to it land, it spoke to me in a language that only I could understand. Watching it land on roof-tops, windows and gathering in gutters creating a stream then disappearing to the pipe and drainage system never to be seen again. Was that to be me? I wondered to myself. My son had his knee operation, it seems successful so glad that it went well for him as it is important for his professional football career. I felt so relieved.

17 April 2012

09:05 hours tablets taken as prescribed. 10:30 hours additional tablets taken as per instructions. Feeling kind of low today, feeling stressed and have a slight pain in right calf. My friend Chris telephoned me today and I informed him of my condition. He suggested lunch at noon and he came over to my home to pick me up and we had a good old chat whilst out at lunch.

18 April 2012

09:10 hours tablets taken as prescribed. 10:40 hours additional tablets taken. Appointment at my local hospital at 17:00 hours today for blood tests which comprises of Renal profile, liver profile, bone profile, PSA level, FBC. Saw my oncologist, received results from PSA reading of 28th of March 2012. PSA reading was 364. Great news, which would suggest that reading taken today, will ultimately be even lower, blood pressure reading 159/83. Vitamin tablets that I had purchased from the store were given approval to take. Any other medication or herbal nutritional tablets have to be approved by my oncologist to ensure that they do not conflict with cancer medication.

I discussed today a list of questions that I had prepared with the doctor. I was informed that I do not need to be admitted at the hospital at any stage unless dire circumstances prevail; also I am not classified as being deemed as terminally ill at present as I am under medication and responding which was good to hear. Doctor suggested that blood spots in my underwear were nothing sinister therefore, nothing to duly concern myself about but it was noted in my file. Radiotherapy treatment of my back not required as yet. However, if back pains do not cease then there is a possibility of this happening. I have to say, elated is not the word, especially the look in the doctors' face at the results made me feel confident that I'm going to beat this cancer, unlike my GPs face when he gave me the news and suggested that I think short-term rather than long-term. I am more than determined to do so now. Grace once again was there with me, can't say how much that meant. She is my angel and my saviour.

I am at home at the moment and the music playing in the background is Laying *Beside me* by soul music band The Isley Brothers a very appropriate song if I may say so. Next appointment is geared up for 2nd May 2012, re-supply of tablets and blood pressure. Called and texted my children and told them the news made me feel good to convey very good news. Stopped in at the Macmillan support office at my local hospital to discuss the benefits. The person responsible won't be in office until Thursday, so I should expect a call to discuss matters.

19 April 2012

06:00 hours, woke up after a restless night, pain in the left hand and arm, pain also in the right elbow area. 09:05 hour tablets taken as prescribed. 11:30 hours additional tablets taken as instructed. Still feeling fatigued, also restarted vitamin tablets. It has become quite clear to me that since the start of the abiraterone tablets, that each week I seem to suffer from one ailment or another which suggests I am undergoing a number of side effect issues. The price one has to pay for treatment I suppose. Contacted Macmillan left message on answer service. Feeling down and depressed if I'm to be honest, not in a good place mentally. Last set of daily tablets taken at 23.00 hours.

20 April 2012

06:15 hours, woke with pain in right leg, calf, and hamstring areas. 09:00 hour tablets taken as prescribed. 11:30 hours additional tablets taken as instructed. Pain still in calf, hamstring areas extending to the foot.
My friend Chris picked me up for lunch at 13:15 hours good to see him again and chat for a few hours and let off some steam. Chris dropped me off in Harrow where my partner lives which saved my partner from taking that long car journey, to pick me up as she normally does

on a Friday for which I am eternally grateful to him. I know Grace was very appreciative of this gesture.

My thoughts are very much seeking answers to the questions of why am I going through the pain on a weekly basis since starting the stampede trials. How much more pain do I have to endure before things settle down? Not nice that I spend weekends at Grace's home and I'm always in pain. What quality of life am I going to have in my last few years if any? As I write my notes, a song on a CD that I compiled is playing. This is the song I want played at my funeral. *Love is Where You Are* by the jazz artist Diana Krall. I have made my daughter Celena aware of this song.

This song is very much dedicated to my partner but also to my children. The words tell where I've been, where I am, and where I'm going. Music has been a key in my life, without which I do not know how I would have coped to be honest. Seems like I'm losing weight, looked in the mirror and I was surprised at what I saw. Not sure I like what I've seen makes me wonder what others are seeing also and not saying. Well, it is fast approaching 23:00 hours time for my MST tablets to be taken. God, I ask that you continue to watch over me, my family, Grace and her family and give me the strength to continue this struggle ahead of me. Without you by my side I cannot do it.

21 April 2012

09:15 hours tablets taken as prescribed. 10:30 hours additional tablets taken as instructed. Still have pain in the calf area of left leg, which is causing me to limp. Relaxed day did not do much at all as my leg hindered me. Called children and updated them on my results from my last appointment. Don't understand this pain that I continue to go through. Only since I've taken the three different tablets that I am regularly going through pain weekly. The extraordinary thing is that it affects different areas of my body and then does not return. Need to discuss in full with doctor at next appointment.

22nd April 2012

I awoke early around 05:15 hours and decide that my partner and I needed to have a heart-to-heart talk. For me the most frustrating change in our sexual relationship has been my loss of libido, "those urges" I used to get frequently are a thing of ancient history. On my part there was no desire to love or be loved sexually and found it very strange for someone like me who has always had a high sex drive. I have begun to lose bodily hair, gained weight, no energy, feeling so tired at times and I certainly hurt in new places in my body. I suppose if I am to be real about it, those issues alone should not surprise me as to why I'm not feeling aroused. More importantly, I do not understand her silent response to the situation that prevails. Grace has not mentioned anything at all about it and as I lay here my mind is working overtime. I am wondering in my mind how she really felt.

As we conversed Grace stated that she had thought about it, but realised that physically that I was not up to it due to the pain I endured in my back, along with the fact that one of the side-effects of the medication was loss of sexual appetite. I still found it hard though to understand that my lifestyle in that direction had evaded me without me really realising, caring about or feeling the loss of, the realisation just crept up on me. Maybe the desire to reengage sexually will come back, but what if it doesn't, I dread the thought.

09:00 hours abiraterone tablets taken as prescribed. 10:15 hours additional tablets taken as instructed. Up and down day due to the left foot and calf plus hamstring hurting, 19:45 hours 1.5 ml of oral morphine taken to combat pain. The pain eased considerably though not totally but none the less easier than earlier. Need to speak with my local hospital on Monday. The pain continued today, so I decided to call the on-call-doctor at my local hospital. I spoke with her and gave her my symptoms she suggested that it could be DVT (deep vein thrombosis) which is a type of blood clot and suggested that I attend

A&E immediately.

My partner Grace drove me there at 22:40 hours upon arrival we explained to reception the situation. I did not realise that a patient in my condition is isolated away from other patients when you enter A&E.

I was seen by a senior staff nurse within 15 minutes. Blood pressure was checked and a reading of 193/94 recorded which was a very high reading, my bloods were taken and expedited for results. I was then seen by the senior house officer and examined thoroughly; bloods came back as showing positive for DVT. An anti-coagulant injection was then administered into my stomach.

Further bloods were taken, arteriolar blood gases right wrist, along with ECG was carried out. My blood pressure was again taken with a new reading recorded as 123/70. Clearly this had dropped dramatically. I was informed that the hospital DVT nurse would call me on Monday afternoon to arrange an ultrasound scan as the doctor wanted to be sure.

Texted my children whilst at the hospital and updated them. My weight was taken and recorded as 121kg. Clearly my blood pressure readings reflect the stress and pain levels that I was undergoing 123/70 indicated the calmness of relaxing in a hospital treatment room without being overly stressed out about life in general. We left the hospital at almost 03:00 hours, I need to contact my oncologist on Monday and update them on my condition and visit to A&E. Once again I am indebted to Grace.

23 April 2012

I awoke at around 07:00 hours still felt very tired from the early morning hospital finish. 09:00 hours tablets taken as prescribed. E-mails sent to research nurse at my local hospital as regards my A&E

visit. I detailed the hospital process and results. 10:00 hours additional tablets taken as instructed. I received a call from the hospital reference an appointment time for ultrasound scan from DVT nurse, which is set for 16:15 hours.

I felt slightly sick after taking the tablets and went back to bed at 14:00 hours for an hour before attending hospital for my appointment. The process was a scan from groin to knee, no clot was found after the scan. It was a great relief to hear this; however, the bone pain is still very much apparent. Apparently false blood readings can occur due to cancer malignant disease. A copy of the report was made available as regards treatment and test undertaken.

I am stressed out at the moment due to some internal family strife which has spilt over into a major altercation. I was not made aware of this as my daughter Lajade did not want me to be stressed out. Upon hearing this I felt helpless and useless in assisting my daughter. A father should be there to protect at all times, but I was not able to do so. Tearful to say the least. Fortunately, though my eldest daughter Celena managed to support her through the issue.

24 April 2012

09:00 hours tablets taken as prescribed. 10:00 hours additional tablets taken as instructed. I realised last night that I had forgotten to take my MST tablets and this morning I felt some pain in the upper thigh area of my right leg and the left side of my back. I really felt very tired yesterday, which is why I probably forgot to take my usual medication hence the early night. Well tears started my day again, I sat on the edge of the bed reflecting on my life and how better a father I could have been and could still be in my remaining time on this earth. Finances preclude me from fulfilling certain things which would make a lot of my concerns go away. I suppose many have similar problems like me and I should be very lucky that I have life at this present stage of my existence.

Financial problems or no financial problems, quality of life is what really matters and I do have that especially with my family and dear friends around me. I am at a loss to understand sometimes as to my lack of fear of dying, but as I have stated on many occasions I feel that I have an angelic being with me. When I get tired as I do, maybe not as I show too often I revert to thinking about God and those dearly departed.

I am indeed continuously grateful to my partner and I feel that I am at times overburdening her with my illness and problems. At times we are at a distance from each other not from the perspective of love, but quality of life. I need to make a firm and final decision as to our partnership as it also affects others. God will guide me in what needs to be done for he has a higher plan for me. Just as I am writing my notes my best friend telephones and I relayed to him the events over the last six days.

A calming effect seems to have come over me, as I realise that some of the things just require me to be patient. It's early days still in the stampede drug trials programme. Clearly the many faces of cancer challenge an individual to show their fighting spirit and will to live, I being one of them.

Pains increased in the left side of my back and around 14:00 hours as I lay prone in bed the pains became so severe that I could not physically move. I knew that I was in trouble, fortunately my mobile phone was next to me and I sent a series of text messages for HELP as I could not move. My partner Grace did not immediately respond, however, my eldest daughter Celena called and I painfully related to her what was occurring she told me that she was calling an ambulance and also contacting the trials nurse at my local hospital. Within minutes the research nurse called me and could hear that I was in a distressed state and told me to call 999 immediately.

Now the drama really starts, I was in such a distressed state that I thought that the house front door was locked. I naturally assume then that the ambulance service or police would have no option but to kick in the door, as I could not locate the front door keys. I knew that there were spare kitchen door and back garden gate keys accessible, but they were in the kitchen. My daughter called my sister who then picked up my daughter from her home, which was about 1 hour drive from my home. Whilst in transit my sister texted me with "Picking up Celena, on our way," A further two text messages are sent that read "Call ambulance they will figure how to get in. This is followed 5 minutes later by another text "get to the hospital".

The next call I receive from my daughter is calm but authoritative and tells me to call the ambulance; however, I am only worried about the damage they will cause to my partner's home in trying to gain access.

I tell my daughter I will try and get up and open the kitchen door and garden gate, she then decides that she will dial 999 for an ambulance. With this in mind, I was still prone in bed, wincing in excruciating pain and unable to move.

But determined I was and determined I became. With phone in hand and my teeth gritted, I slide my body off the bed onto the floor. I then managed to get onto my knees and push back on my legs (like as if I was in a push up position) and used my hands to push myself up and away from the bed into an upright position. The pain was unbelievable as I pushed and stood up shakily. With this achieved I then pigeon stepped to the kitchen where I located the relevant keys, but, before I could reach the kitchen door into the garden I collapsed three times onto the kitchen marble floor.

Each time having to lift myself up again into the erect vertical walking position. The pain was now blowing my mind away, I could not cry, I was beyond tears, I just gritted my teeth harder and focused on reaching the kitchen door. I recalled a great sigh upon reaching the first door, but knew I had another at a greater distance away to get too.

What would usually take me ordinarily a round trip of 40 seconds took me about 9 minutes. Left, Right, Left, Right, Left, Right, that's how I did it to blank out the pain from my mind. Having achieved this feat I returned to my bedroom to await the ambulance persons. I remember trying to call Grace again on her cell phone, but without any luck. Where was she when I needed her most, I had become so reliant on this woman and now she was nowhere to be found. Had something happened to her, I had thought, my mind was all over the place and panic was trying and in fact had gotten a hold of me. As I lay prone the only thought that entered my mind, was what if a burglar entered our property now, I would have been useless and unable to defend the property. The moment for prayer beckoned and in my mind, I recited the Lord's Prayer.

As I waited for the ambulance to arrive the pain became increasingly un-bearable and at that moment I was finding it hard to breathe. Each deep breath I took seemed to cause more pain in my back. I had already taken 1.5 ml, of oral morph medication for the break through pain but this had not worked.

My partner Grace then called and informed me she was on her way from work to home, at that present moment in time she was in the town of Bushey which was only about 15 minutes away, I got mad with her which was so wrong of me as I had tried several times to get her but could not get her, as it turned out it was a simple case of she had been in a meeting with phone switched off, I raged to be honest but then I realised that the pain had placed me into a state of confusion and totally unreasonable behaviour.

I recall hearing in the distance an ambulance siren whilst I lay in bed but, it just remained a distant sound as the pain over took me. This was the original pain coming back that had started the ball rolling in 2011 and as we know now this was the pain called cancer running through my body.

The pain had now reached a level that I had never reached before and all I could do was to continue gritting my teeth and hang in there. Prayer was no longer a viable option I was past concentrating on God, at which the front door bell rang and then again, and then again. I just knew that it was the ambulance crew, and hoped to god it was not a parcel mail delivery. But if it was them then somehow the message had not been passed to them to 'Go around the back of the property, the gate was open as the front door was locked.' The bell ringing continued and once again I had to contort and twist my body which responded with burning pain and make my way now to the front door, (fortunately for me the property was a ground floor flat so no stairs). I had surpassed myself; I had physically done something that for which they normally pin medals on your chest for. Upon reaching the front door which was glass plated I saw a male para-medic standing there on his radio, I mentally noted the few words 'please cancel the police unit looks like we do not need to gain access again.' I could not talk I was voiceless and not one word could I utter and he noted me gesturing with my left hand to go around the side to the garden door and gain access to the house that way.

At this point all I could do was to prop myself up against the front door frame as I was void of energy all had been used up. I had nothing left to give or anywhere to go but on the floor, I was out on my feet totally exhausted after giving it my all. Within seconds the ambulance crew entered the property just in time as I was about to collapse, luckily for me one of the crew was over 6ft and fairly well built. I recall him saying just rest against me mate, we will get you a chair were his words. His partner a blonde female took a chair from the front lounge and made me sit on it. I recall just slouching onto the chair and then the questions started to flow from them barely audible to me as the pain had silenced everything.

I think I only answered two or three before the front door opened and there stood my Angel Grace who looked down at me sitting in the chair. Her face contorted with the look of flustered panic.

I recalled her almost in tears before the male ambulance crew member told her to calm down before he had to take the two of us in the ambulance. From this moment on Grace took over the questions and direction of my care. I was given some funny gas to inhale which I have to say worked a treat but I remember Grace telling me afterwards when she opened the front door and observed me in the chair, that I looked very white in fact bloodless, like all the life had been drawn out of me. Little did she realise how true that could have been for I felt that I was not far from meeting my creator. I recall the ambulance crew wanting to get a chair to wheel me into ambulance but I was defiant and told them I would walk, in reality that day a tortoise would have got their quicker but the crew were very patient and understanding.

Upon entering the ambulance I was given more gas and felt the pain easing and felt very light headed a light high I would describe it as.

Grace followed in her car to our local hospital where I was taken. I recalled being wheeled in and Lajade my daughter waiting there with a worried expression on her face. Now I was surrounded by two loved ones, where an hour ago I had no one. The unabated excitement that was felt was priceless. At this point in my mind if I had died I would have died happily.

I was placed in a cubical with partner and my younger daughter Lajade by my side. I remember asking where Celena my eldest was as I knew she was on her way and would hold everything together where the children were concerned. Lajade had that fish out of water look and that wasn't going to help neither her nor me.

Lajade informed me she was in contact via text messaging with her and she and my sister were en-route to the hospital. The gas had now worn off and the pain was coming back, now with a vengeance.

The A&E nurse administered further morphine intravenously, in total

35 mg was given to me and in the short term nothing worked. I vividly recall noting that Celena and my sister Valentina had arrived and was in the cubical with us, I now had four women around me, what a lucky fella I was. The pain had now reached an eleven out of ten. All who were around me were in tears as I clutched the hospital bed rail and moaned, groaned, jerked and twitched in severe pain. Their voices I heard asking the nurse and doctor to do something for the pain (my eyes welt as I recall the moment). This reminded me of October 2011, when I attended A&E at for a similar pain I really thought after that episode that no one would ever see me in pain like this again. This was not to be the case I really felt for all and my tears were a combination of pain and sadness for what they were undergoing more than for myself. It took almost four hours from admission for the A&E team to bring my pain down to a moderate level.

It was decided that whilst I was still in pain that I would be admitted to hospital for further, observation and tests. Subsequently I was transferred to an AAU ward (Acute Assessment Unit) at around 23.45 hours whereupon my family departed and I was now left on my own once again. At 01.00 hours I was then transferred to another ward which was to be my temporary home for the next 4 days. An uneventful hospital stay was far from what happened next, this crazy event that took place was like something out of a movie, at first I thought that maybe the morphine was playing mind games with me. At around 03:00 hours whilst propped up in my bed and floating in and out of sleep, I noticed a person pass on the opposite side of the ward and enter into a bed bay area and pull the curtains around the bed.

Though somewhat groggy I assumed that this was a nurse or doctor examining a patient and I fell back into a sleep. I don't know how long I was asleep for before being woken to the sounds of loud voices especially that of one of the female nurses. It turned out that the person whom I had seen walk across into the bay bed area was a female intruder and worst still had gotten into an empty bed and was asleep before the nursing staff realised that she was an intruder. I recall the conversation as the intruder stated she was a patient (however with no wristband) but I could see she was fully clothed in civilian clothing though scruffy. For a few minutes a conversation flowed as she insisted she was a patient and the nursing staff telling her she could not be, especially as there was a policy for no female patients on a male ward.

I could hear the irateness in the nurses' voices and then it became pungently clear why as a whiff came across my nostrils of urine. She had pissed the bed up. With the threat of security being called, the intruder walked off the ward and I took it she was escorted off the unit section. I remember saying to the male nurse that she had a cheek, he replied yes, however, she had left them all a present that had be cleaned up. With that, the mattress was removed and a new mattress was bought in and the area thoroughly cleaned.

In my afterthought analysis, the frightening thought of having my throat cut became clear to me, how did she get into the ward, as to gain access you have to press a buzzer and be electronically admitted. Not until I left the ward to go home before I realised that there was a flaw…The doors open out when opening and are on a slow release open and shut timer and unless someone is actually physically or visually monitoring the admission of someone to the ward area it was easy for someone to gain access and even hide in a toilet or cupboard area before moving further into the ward. Hopefully the report made by the staff was acted upon and some solution made by the security department. The following morning I found out that she was a person living rough on the streets and needed somewhere warm to stay for the night.

25 April 2012

The hospital, attended to my medical care and I was very tired today, as I had, not had a good night's sleep due to an eventful early morning aforementioned escapade. 06:00 hours blood pressure taken recorded reading was 131/70, blood sugar taken recorded reading 9.8ng/ml. Later that morning at 09:00 hours blood pressure taken reading recorded as 141/83. My usual tablets which were left by my partner Grace were given to me and I took as per usual instructions. The consultant came to see me on the ward and examined me and referred me for an MRI scan along with an investigation of my bladder as the A&E x-ray had shown lots of gas. My blood sugar reading was taken again at 11:36 hours recorded reading showed 11.4ng/ml

I urinated in the urinal bowel by my bedside as I finished my back just gave way and I collapsed back onto the bed in pain. Whatever is going on had not finished. Seems like I may have to stay another day in the hospital due to more tests required, I was not happy about this at all, I just wanted to go home and be cared for by my partner.

13:50 hours blood pressure taken recorded reading 140/80 MST 30 mg also administered. Felt very lonely this morning, the sun came out late morning after a dreary morning, but no one came to visit me, as they had promised, felt very low after yesterday's painful admission.

Still felt sick to my stomach, the excess morphine taken yesterday still played up on me. Doctor requested my previous MRI scans from St. Mary's Hospital in Paddington, London, where I originally had my scan carried out, as this they say will help them to compare a then and now scan. 17:55 hours blood pressure taken recorded reading 149/70, which prompted the visitors to start coming. Firstly, my baby sister Doreen, my daughter Lajade, my partner Grace and my best friend Tosin. Felt better that I had some family and friends in my corner though; I looked drained in my face and also felt very tired.

I need to make contact with my oncologist as I am a little confused with certain questions and procedures that were carried out at the A&E department of the hospital that I am admitted to. My sister,

Valentina texted me it read "Just remember he neither sleeps nor slumbers, he continues to watch over you even when others have gone. His faithfulness is everlasting to all who call upon him".

26 April 2012

Alarm set for 01:30 hours as the nurse needs to give me my MST. Argued with the nurse about her reluctance to give me my MST. Angry was not the word, I insisted that my medication be given and this only occurred after senior nurse intervened and agreed. 01:45 hours MST given I intend to make a complaint to the doctor later today. Blood pressure taken at 06:00 hours readings 129/78, blood sugar taken at 06:46 hours reading 5.2. At 08:40 hours abiraterone tablets taken as prescribed. Additional tablets taken an hour later.

Grace texted me it read "I feel we have got so much closer over the past few months and share something special. I need you to know I am here for you and my love for you grows every day (made me feel special and a great start to the day). 08:44 hours bloods were taken by nurses. Stomach feels woozy and I am going through a hot flush moment. Just want to go home now fed up with being cooped up and feeling like no one cares or loves me.

At this present moment in time my back feels fine. Just a few minor pains, but nothing compared to yesterday.

The ward that I am on now is primarily for cancer patients. A gentleman called Steve is in the bed next to me and introduced himself and we started to have an interesting chat I really was impressed by him and the conversation we had.

I whinge and moan at times, but here's a guy in his sixty's who has it far worse than me with his femur eaten out by cancer and he required pins to keep his lower body area intact. Bubbly, polite, well travelled, with maybe five or so years to live, but with an attitude I envied.

I always believed that God puts positive people in our way when we least expect it. As I looked into his face and eyes I could see a guy who had accepted his fate and destiny.

Right there and then the colour of skin was not a barrier for our dialogue just two grown adult men talking about life in general and forgetting for a moment about our ailments. I did not instigate this conversation, but felt after forty five minutes that I had known this man all my life.

A smile was on my face with the guy all the time. 10:19 hours blood pressure taken 139/83, temperature 36.6, heart rate 78. Doctor, examined me checked all the usual things plus spine, legs, foot, stated that MRI scan that I was to undergo could be today or tomorrow. Once they have done this and controlled the pain, then I would be discharged and allowed to go home. Follow-up care will then be carried out by my local hospital oncology department. Doctor has requested that I remain in bed to alleviate pressure on my back.

Visitors galore today, my daughters Lajade and Celena, a good friend of mine, Chris, my partner Grace and my sisters along with Church pastor Steven Ramos, who spent a considerable amount of time with me. Pastor Ramos said an encouraging prayer of power today at my bedside which came with the word from God that I will beat this cancer. For me though the best part of the day was having father and daughter time, which was so meaningful to me, those reading this book with children will understand fully the feeling.

I officially introduced Grace to my daughters as my partner in our one-to-one chat. No problem there whatsoever, especially Lajade she took to the news very well. Celena well, she's a harder nut to crack and nodded in approval, but with a reserved demeanour which said time will tell dad, time will tell.

In my heart though, I knew that I was with the right person, soul mate and lifelong partner all rolled up into one. Emotionally, though I was all over the place here I was now with the right partner, but facing a death sentence maybe sooner or maybe later I knew not. The main question that lay with me was why Grace would want to stay with someone in my condition, maybe the fact that she had a medical background had something to do with it, but also maybe she saw qualities and traits that appealed to her that overruled my current condition.

Had a visit from the Macmillan urology Cancer nurse which was rather unexpected but perfect as I had a complaint to lay at her door. I explained to her the lack of response from my local hospital Macmillan office.

Also discussed with her my current care under my local hospital and stampede drug trial to date. Interesting response came from her that I may have to reconsider coming off the trial programme should the pain continue as she said not all trial programmes are always suitable for everyone. 15:00 hours MRI scan undertaken which lasted for forty minutes spinal cord, lower and upper back, scanned, results will be available tomorrow and then hopefully I will be discharged. In myself, I still did not feel 100% perfect along with an uneasy feeling in general.

Steve in bed next to me still continues to inspire me and reassure me, for this I will always be eternally grateful. Contacted research nurse with updates, she suggested that I may have to see a consultant on the 2nd May now due to my hospitalisation.

21:45 hours blood pressure reading was 146/84. My two daughters who were present for most of this week Lajade and Celena represent the best part of my life. They showed love, courage and determination along with leadership. They made me so proud of them without a doubt. No father could ask for more, but I did and I got more as tears blur my vision as I write my heart rejoices in these two daughters. Thank you God, thank you. A nurse administered an Anti-DVT injection in my stomach due to lack of physical movement and bed restriction whilst in hospital.

27 April 2012

06:00 hours blood pressure reading 132/86, blood sugar level 5.8, temperature 37. Feeling in myself better, except my stomach, but that is due to laxatives taken and is to be expected but no bowel movement currently. 09:30 hours doctor visited and discussed details of MRI scan, negative findings, no compression on spine found other than large deposits of metastases on spine.

In comparison to the previous MRI scan taken all seems to be stable. They cannot explain the reason why flare-up occurred other than the large metastatic deposits in my spine area. The possibility of this happening again is realistic though and I wonder to myself can my heart take such a strain on it again, regardless of the fact that I have a good healthy heart. Discharge of myself was approved, however PSA test needed to be carried out before I am discharged. All details are to be forwarded to oncology department where I was receiving my care for them to carry out further investigation. Blood pressure reading of 145/88 and temperature 36.9 recorded.

Requested prescription for new MST tablets in 15mg formula as my current formula is 10 mg. Glad that I'm going home as I was getting very depressed in my surroundings. Found out that the guy in the bed next to me on the right side is heading for a hospice, I overheard a conversation between him and doctors which scared me no end. He was not totally happy in going into a hospice. I heard him refer to a friend who had gone into a hospice and lasted four days before passing away. I would tend to agree with him to go home. Well discharge time came around 13:00 hours and I said goodbye to two patients and the medical team.

Did not say goodbye to Steve as he was not in his bed when I was discharged, but I intended to go back and see him before I leave Harrow and head home. Steve was placed there for a reason and we have not said our farewells yet. Grace picked me up and we came home, it is a lovely feeling to be home and felt love and support again, not that I was not getting it, though just that hospital environment differ greatly from home.

Still weak on my feet, clearly due to lack of movement over the three-day hospitalisation. Bags of medication given which confuse the hell out of me will consult staff at appointment   next week but will take prescribed MST.

My body and mind were very tired, so I decided to get some sleep. I immediately went to sleep and slept solidly for three hours, even phone calls and text messages did not disturb my sleep. I awoke for about thirty minutes, then fell back to sleep for about another five to six hours. It is now 01:10 hours as I make my notes, felt slightly tired but generally well in body.

Read my hospital discharge letter in full and noted the comparisons made from 15 January 2012, MRI scan stating stable except pelvic adenopathy though stable, there is metastatic deposits seen in the C3 vertebral body L2 L3, L5, S2 and S3. No evidence of extra osseous spread and no evidence of compression of the spinal Canal. I am without a doubt worried about my condition and that I could have a repeat of the lumbar pain, without a doubt a chronic pain that on a scale of one to ten rates fifteen. Every movement I made or every step I took was one step closer to that pain returning and the issue here was now one of pain management control and should I have another attack it is my firm wish that my family do not witness this.

I have learnt so much about myself this week as I have about others who are affected by the disease. Just realised that I made a note on the 2nd April 2012, which really prepared me inadvertently with regards to a cancer ward visitation at my local hospital. Not realising that, that visit was preparing me for the week that I have had. Very strange set of events this week, however, I had been unknowingly prepared for this.

Anybody of a lesser physical stature and strength or weaker would have given up after what I endued is my belief. But what lies ahead requires more than strength, it requires faith and love of thyself and family. My daughters Lajade and Kira have both changed because of this at a time in their life when they both needed it. Celena showed leadership love and hope. It is only because of the distance that Kira is unable to be by my side more often, but her text messages and phone calls make up for her absence as they convey all the love she has for her father.

28 April 2012

09:15 hours abiraterone tablets taken as described. 10:45 hours additional tablets taken along with 30 mg of MST. Still feel groggy in head and stomach. No pain in back area, though, throughout the day felt twinges in various parts of the body but nothing sinister. Showered as I felt clammy and dirty, felt real good after and made sure all my clothes from the hospital were washed along with home bedding slept on last night.

Just wanted to create a distance between then and now. It drizzled most of the day so could not get out for a walk, maybe Sunday will yield better weather.

Back pain returned in the area of my right hip, I have stiffness in my left foot that caused me to limp around. I have made tentative arrangements with my daughter Celena and my partner Grace should this happen again as to what they are to do. 11:30 hours MST taken 30 mg along with two sachets of Macrogol compound powder.

Felt twinges in back still carefully monitoring these pains. Plan in place should I need to go back to the hospital. Concern is growing amongst my daughters as my constant pain as revealed to me tonight in a phone conversation my sister Pat who had called me stated 'Your daughters are hurting she said.'

But I am fully aware of this and had my sister been more of a sister than a gas bag then she would have known. I have issues with some members of my family who show two different faces neither conducive to my betterment, they just add to the stress. I am aware that my children are feeling the pain and maybe the answer is to try and show a different face if I can but, when you have metastatic cancer bone pain it's unlike any pain I have ever known, and hiding it just is not at all humanly possible.

29 April 2012

09:00 hours abiraterone tablets taken as prescribed. 10:30 hours. additional tablets taken as instructed. Felt good today, no real pain as such though, still somewhat unsteady on my feet especially during my morning shower. Had a heart-to-heart talk with Grace today as it is Sunday morning felt we had reached a milestone in our relationship which was reciprocated by her and greatly appreciated by me.

It has taken our relationship up ten notches. Decided to get an early night as body and mind are tired, having gone for a walk earlier today which was tiring. Last of medication taken at 22.00 hours.

30th April 2012

01:40 hours woke with sharp pains from groin upwards to which I arched my back in response; pain lasted for about thirty seconds. 09:00 hours abiraterone tablets taken as prescribed. Contacted hospital to confirm the consultation appointment, which had been made for Wednesday 2nd May 2012, at 17:00 hours. 11:15 hours took additional tablets as instructed. Feeling stressed as it's a new week and personal finances are depleted and matters are dire. I have no idea what I'm going to do.

It's very hard to smile sometimes in life, there are things that happen that you don't understand and you don't know if you are going to get through it.

I'm going through storms in my life right now that I don't know how long they will last. Still a few pains were felt throughout the day. Spoke with hospital who now require me to come in tomorrow at 11:00 hours for blood and blood pressure tests.

Time-consuming this is becoming in more ways than one. Started the new morphine sulphate 10 mg slow release tablets, felt very woozy after taking them.

Had a few bowel movements throughout the day, which eased the blockage in my stomach area which was making me feel further unwell. Early to bed tonight as I have a busy day on Tuesday. One thing is for sure a lot of quality time is being spent with Grace, who has given me a lot of hope and joy.

One month of treatment has now passed and I was doing well, besides the hospitalisation blip, I was doing wonderfully well. Abiraterone had lived up to its reviews and I was a living testimony of this. Yes the side effects were very uncomfortable but I knew this was the price one had to pay to stay alive. At this stage now I am on the internet, carrying out a little research. I had told myself previously to stay away from it as it's a minefield of misinformation as well as information. I knew that I was in a serious risk category which in combination with my GP's previous statement 'think short term rather than long term' a niggling desire for correctness was echoing in my head and I need clarity and confirmation. As an Afro Caribbean male I was in the high risk group and further information researched suggested more: -

"Who is at risk?

In the UK, about one in eight men will get prostate cancer at some point in their lives. Older men, men with a family history of prostate cancer and Black men are more at risk.

Age

Prostate cancer mainly affects men over the age of fifty and your risk increases with age. The average age for men to be diagnosed with prostate cancer is between seventy and seventy four years. If you are under fifty then your risk of getting prostate cancer is very low. Younger men can be affected, but this is rare.

Family history

You are two and a half times more likely to get prostate cancer if your father or brother has been diagnosed with it, compared to a man that has no relatives with prostate cancer. You may have a higher risk of prostate cancer if your mother or sister has had breast cancer, particularly if they were diagnosed under the age of sixty.

Black men

Black men are more likely to get prostate cancer than men of other ethnic backgrounds. In the UK, about 1 in 4 Black men will get prostate cancer at some point in their lives. The reasons for this are not yet clear, but might be linked to genes.

Lifestyle

No one knows how to prevent prostate cancer, but diet and a healthy lifestyle may be important in "protecting against the disease".

Information sourced from: -
http://prostatecanceruk.org/information/who-is-at-risk

It's shocking to know that one in four black men in the UK will be diagnosed with prostate cancer at some point in their lifetime. That's double the overall one-in-eight cradle to grave risk faced by all men in the UK. Russian roulette springs to mind, but in this scenario four players are chancing the bullet. Four - Five years could easily pass before I would visit my GP. However, if I am to be outright honest, my GP a supposed trained professional missed screening me, especially as my family history is fraught with cancer deaths.

But as I have said I was never the first in line to see a GP, I tended to shy away from my rights to health care whether from a GP point of view or helpline. The heightened cancer risk that was clearly before me, I failed to engage and take the necessary preventive corrective actions.

During this first month of treatment I felt at times it was becoming confusing to differentiate between the drug side effects and my prostate cancer symptoms. Evidently all drugs used to treat cancer cause side effects. Side effects are unwanted things that can happen to you as a direct result of medical treatment – in my case, taking a cancer treatment drug such as abiraterone or hormone injection such as Prostap.

The varying pains throughout my body at times suggested to me that it was the cancer, but during consultation appointments it was suggested by my doctors that these were indeed side effects, though at times I was not fully convinced that the doctors knew exactly if that was the case. The term clutching at straws sprung to mind on many occasions, especially as I was on a medical trial programme.

I was fearful of the fact that I was a guinea pig in a new medical trial programme which to me meant they the doctors didn't know or have all the answers and as such trying to find those answers myself via the internet was an impossible feat. Fortunately, my partner was on hand to back up a lot of my symptom complaints as she lay next to me at night she heard and saw the reaction to pain, twinges, jerks and more. Grace being an NHS employee gave way to an experienced and qualified medical person to give additional support at my consultation appointments.

The pains I was subjected to were not just any ordinary pains these bordered on chronic pains and took pain to a different level at times. I recall Grace looking at me tearfully on numerous occasions in total shock and disbelief at the pain I was undergoing. What she didn't know was the pain I underwent during the day when she was at work and I was at home by myself. Very rarely during this first month did my children see me in pain, tears maybe but pain I intentionally hide from them

For now what was working was the medication even to the surprise of the doctors, I quote a remark in a report "I was delighted to meet Mr. Samuels today. His presenting PSA was 500 and his most recent PSA today is 2.4. He has had an excellent PSA response with abiraterone and hormones and we hope that this continues.

He tells me, he feels low in mood, low energy levels and these are almost certainly related to his low testosterone levels, which are artificially generating with our LHRH analogue. This is unfortunately something that he may have to put up with as a reward for PSA control".

This report extract for me precisely summarised what was medically going on within me during this period. , My mental state was something above and beyond the usual stresses of everyday life, and the experience of a whole range of emotions and feelings such as pain, fear, anger, sadness, guilt, chemical castration and disbelief.

Stress was at the forefront of many of my low days during this first month of treatment caused by many things, including work, money worries other health concerns such as diabetes Type 11. I began to realise that everyone reacts differently to stress and there was no right or wrong way to deal with it, other than I could not let any chinks in my armour be found.

Work for me was an escape from my diagnosis, but that meant stress. You cannot run a business without stress being a part of your day. As I saw it, everything was about swings and roundabouts, I can attest to that. If I could just close everything down without penalties and relax for a few months, then that would be the answer to my personal situation, but I was the sole proprietor without any keyman insurance a detrimental business error on my side.

I have for the past few months been feeling very guilty about contracting the disease and with a family cancer history, such as mine, I questioned how I let slip this crucial and very important check up. I recall having personal thoughts about this over the years and my GP suggesting that after the age of fifty, that I should have regular checkups. Work and life just seemed to take precedence and the checks were not carried out and now I am paying the price. I knew that the PSA test, which could give me an early indication of prostate cancer, was available to me, but I failed to act upon it. As the years have passed, I have carried out a little research only to find out that experts disagree on how useful the PSA test is. To date in the United Kingdom there still is no national screening programme for Afro Caribbean males as relates prostate cancer.

1 May 2012

07:30 hours abiraterone tablets taken as described. 08:45 hours additional tablets taken as instructed. Attended local hospital for bloods and blood pressure taken reading of 154/89 at 11:30 hours. For the first time since making notes I read back some of what I've written to Grace and it impacted on her quite emotionally. I really did it to gauge the strength of what I was writing and how my nearest and dearest were feeling about what I had suffered. Equally to share some of my inner thoughts and emotions with her, which she appreciated.

I have noticed that my urge to urinate frequently was becoming lesser and lesser. Also, my weepish moments due to the hormone injection were also, seemingly, under control. Actually, there are moments of late that I feel that I am free of this disease and there are times when I jump up without restriction to any bodily part or I walk very quickly to people's amazement and mine when it is revealed to me.

Stopped by the Macmillan nurse's office and discussed application form with a Citizen Advice Bureau advisor, again, not sure totally that what he is saying is relevant and maybe a call to original phone representative is needed as there is a reluctance to step on the toes of my original representative. Relaxing evening and felt fairly good no real aches and pains. Early night as I have a long day again on Wednesday, last of my daily medication taken at 23:15 hours.

2 May 2012

09:00 hours abiraterone tablets taken as described. 10:05 hours additional tablets taken as instructed with breakfast. After a shower and towelling off and then clothing I felt extremely tired and felt that my energy levels were totally sapped. This really was a first and once again something else to ponder on, though I have to understand fatigue is a major part of cancer and maybe this is what I was undergoing. Had a bowel movement earlier today, though it was small nonetheless a movement which done me the world of good, as I had felt my bowel system was becoming clogged up.

Realising more and more that I am heavily reliant on my partner and do not feel comfortable with this at all. I am so use to being self-reliant and now that has all changed. Our relationship is moving onwards and upwards and I am frightened by the notion of my disease becoming a major barrier, and her moving on. This is not a lifestyle for the faint hearted or the usual, but then again Grace is not the usual, far from it.

We all have our needs, needs that I cannot right now provide for and maybe in the long term permanently unable to give. All of these things play havoc with my mind on a daily basis, not because I don't write everything down, that it doesn't mean it's not there, it most definitely is.

Why me Lord, why me, I ask every day, especially when I have found somebody very special, who I believed to be my lifelong partner. A few people walked in and out of my life, but only one true love has left a footprint in my heart like she has. There are many an occasion that I thought that the doctors could have got it wrong and I hoped for a miraculous reversal, of their diagnosis, but as each day passes it has begun to register that it was here and here to stay for now. The half smiles I have seen on their faces gave it all away; after all they are only but human aren't they?

Appointment with Registrar at 15:30 hours, which I attended with Grace, explained the events leading up to my recent hospital admission and the care received. The doctor referred to the MRI scan taken whilst I was admitted. He went through the x-ray, which showed the affected cancer areas on the scan. The main areas showing up were the lower back and groin areas, it was clear to me that what I was seeing were all the areas that I had been complaining about. The doctor suggested that I may need radiotherapy treatment, combined with orthopaedic surgery on my back byways of a cement type substance being injected into my vertebra which, would assist in the overall radiotherapy treatment.

The radiotherapy treatment would consist of treatment, once-a-day for five days and he believed that the procedures should be carried out within the next two months. With this in mind, I clearly was about to undergo an onslaught of treatment in a limited time frame. Effectively, this would help reduce the pain that I have undergone. If I do not have the operation, then the pain could continue.

How much more do I have to go through and more importantly, how much more, does my family have to endure? Mentally the feeling of undergoing this kind of operation did not rest well with me; I just had a feeling that this was a mistake in the making. The one big bit of news was that my PSA level taken on the 1st May 2012, registered 254, which showed that the tablets are working. Big smile on my face as the thoughts going through my head over the past few weeks were, that the tablets were the fault, now clearly this thought has been laid to rest.

A new appointment is arranged for 30 May 2012, to manage further the proposed operation and radiotherapy treatment. I text messaged my family immediately, to advise them of the proposed treatment and alleviate current worries.

Obtained from oncology department new abiraterone tablets 2 x 120 tablet bottles along with prednisolone 5mg tablets x 30. A new appointment was made for 31 May 2012 at 16:00 hours, at the Trevor Howell ward. The next few weeks and months are going to test my strength, patience, endurance and will to live to the maximum, well early night again 23:00 hours.

3 May 2012

09:00 hours abiraterone tablets taken as prescribed. 10:15 hours additional tablets taken as instructed. Felt fairly good today, no real pain as such. Grace investigated medical procedures for radiotherapy treatment, along with the orthopaedic operation. The information returned suggests that it will be quite a lay off for me, with possible side effects of up to two years in the making. Lajade my daughter came over and spent the day with Grace and me. As is always the case my diamond daughter shines out always and a smile was on my face for the remainder of the day. The back pain has resurfaced again, complied with doctors recommendation of extra ibuprofen and paracetamol tablets.

4 May 2012

09:00 hours abiraterone tablets taken as prescribed. 10:30 hours additional tablets taken as instructed, vitamin tablets also taken. Felt fairly good this morning, no real pain to complain about. I went for a walk in the local park today, to exercise my leg muscles which felt real good. One of my physical problems is that I am not exercising my joint muscles enough; as I remain housebound for most of the week other than the hospital appointments I attend. Therefore, as such I am cramping and stiffening up during these lax periods.

Returned to hospital to see Steve, we had a brief chat to say our final goodbyes. I really felt good in myself for doing this, as it was something that I felt I wanted and needed to do, even though I did not really know this person. Our conversations during the time I was admitted meant a lot to me, in the face of adversity and disability, he had shown me that others are far worse off than me, what an upbeat guy. I know he appreciated the visit though; he was going home this weekend he still showed true grit and determination. Whilst I was there the physiotherapist was putting him through his paces with crutches and stairs to negotiate he was made to push himself and accomplish. I watched with admiration as he went up and down a number of times using the crutches. What a sight.

We said our goodbyes and shook hands and I departed knowing I would probably never see this man again, but an impact had been made and left in my mind to always remember him by.

Spoke online via Skype today with a client Lt.Colonel Garcia from Trinidad and Tobago government who I have now revealed my condition too. He expressed wishes for a full recovery, stating that his father had, undergone prostate cancer for over twenty years and now aged seventy five was still very much alive and well. So he was able to sympathise with me for my condition. He suggested a plant called saw palmetto, available in health food shops an excellent product on all accounts. Also suggested 100 mg of zinc an herbal treatment. As he is due in the UK on May 18th, he proposed bringing along some helpful remedies with him and some expert advice from some cancer consultant friends based in Trinidad. All the help and assistance was most welcome is what I thought. Though he was a client, we had developed a friendly but professional relationship in the short time we had known each other.

Still being stressed by some family issues concerning my daughters. Looks like I have to intervene so as not to see my children end up in trouble. I cannot as their father allow anything to happen to them and sit back and be comfortable about not doing anything. Delicate as the matter is, it does however mean a kid gloves approach, plus cleverness and diplomacy need to be used. As the evenings draw in my back just seems to get stiffer, even though the central heating is on full blast.

Tonight I read some more of my journal to Grace, to whom I am still growing very, very close to. She listened with empathy to my narration and I to her invaluable response. A tear I saw and then another and another fell from her cheek onto the bedcovers. It is never my deliberate intention to make her cry; I just wanted and needed to share some more of my thoughts. I continued to read to her not for a sadistic reason, but for no other purpose than to show my love for her which were echoed in the narration which were all about her part in my care.

After a few verses I stopped and checked and there she was with those lovely warm brown piercing eyes, sending out vibes of love at me. Enough I said to her, maybe again in a few months' time I'll share some more and we drifted off to sleep with the aforementioned thoughts and words on our minds for our dreams.

5 May 2012

09:00 hours abiraterone tablets taken as instructed 11:00 hours additional tablets taken as prescribed. It is now over a month since I've been taking the abiraterone tablets and I have had mixed feelings throughout this time. There are times that I felt that I should come off the stampede drug trials as I felt that it was not effective and or, causing me more problems than I desire. Clearly the results are proving me wrong and I intend to pursue the programme until the end of the trials. Today I feel a little woozy and unsteady on my feet, other than that I am fine. Went for a walk in local park.

6 May 2012

09:00 hours abiraterone tablets taken as prescribed 10:30 hours additional tablets taken as instructed. Woke today with no real pains or aches, started packing my travel bag and returned home to Surrey after almost 2 weeks of being a guest at Grace's home. I'm going to miss her and her home, but I am well enough to return to my own home. Neither do I wish to overstay my welcome, though this was never an issue. She has been terrific throughout: caring, considerate, loving, and attentive to all my needs and more.

I don't know what I can say or do, to tell her what this has meant to me, but I'll find a way to show her for sure I will.

It's going to be like Adam without his rib Eve, but like I said time to go home and sort out my own personal affairs. I had Sunday dinner at my daughter's home, it was great home cooking. Had another of our heart-to-heart talks tonight, about a wide range of personal matters affecting the family. Felt really good that we spoke and it cleared my mind, of certain fears and concerns that I was having about my family.

I felt very tearful at times and fought hard not to cry though, my daughter sensed it was coming on, I managed to hold off. My sister Tina, who resides in the USA, telephoned whilst I was at my daughter's and we discussed my current medical issues. If I have not previously stated then let me do so now, my sister who is older than me is the assistant director of nursing at the M. D. Anderson Cancer Centre Hospital in Houston, Texas, United States of America.

As such she deals with cancer patients and cancer on a daily basis. Her advice I seek a great deal at the moment as I go through my cancer pain and treatment. She requested that I pass on to her my biopsy results which should reveal the tumour staging. She had discussed matters with a consultant there who was unhappy that I was on the stampede drug trials programme and that I should only have gone on it after the failure of the first hormone treatments.

I attempted to explain to her why I was on the stampede trials at this present moment in time and that I was actually doing quite well, in that my PSA levels were falling and at this particular moment in time it was recorded in 254. It was also suggested that I should start receiving radiotherapy for the pain in my back. Again, I informed her that this was on the cards to be done over the next few weeks.

She suggested that I keep an eye on my blood pressure, making sure that it was kept around and below 130/80.

Grace passed on the following as regards the blood sugar level before meals, reading between four to seven and two hours after eating under 8.5 One thing for sure is that the American way of treating cancer patients does differ to UK.

I had to be careful in seeing and understanding that regardless of the fact that she is my sister, as well as the thousands of miles that we are adrift, as opposed to my consultants who were a few miles from my residency.

7 May 2012

09:00 hours abiraterone tablets taken as prescribed. 12:30 hours additional tablets taken as instructed a little late though, but generally having no impact on me feeling fairly well today, no real pain. First night back at home, felt lost, no Grace there, especially in the morning barking out reminders to me about tablets or what did I want as a cooked breakfast, oh well back to reality for sure. My daughter Celena took me out today to pizza express. It was great spending some quality time with her and also being cheered up by her.

She always has a knack of lifting my spirits, when they are down. Asked my daughter the delicate question of whom she had confided in her dad's ailment, to which she responded only her close friend and an old girlfriend of mine. Only really wanted to know, so that I could try and understand how my daughter was feeling, coping and dealing with the issue at hand.

Tough she maybe as love beams from her face, but more importantly from her heart also. Getting used to doing things for myself again is still a bit of a strange feeling, actually for both Grace and me. Today she informed me she played her music extremely loud at her home something she does not usually do, in fact not at all. For this act she got a visit from the local noise abatement unit as a neighbour complained. Of course, I got the blame, smile. 8 May 201209:00 hours abiraterone tablets taken as described. 10:50 hours additional tablets taken as instructed. Today I felt relaxed with no real pain, decided to drop off Macmillan grant forms at my GP for medical reports. Can't really say how I feel mentally other than not in pain and not stressed, nor am I emotional a rare day for sure.

Spoke with Grace today for one hour, five minutes where we had another of our deep heart-to-heart conversations which actually went deeper than at any time before. She spoke of her fear of us splitting up and felt reassured from our conversation that, this was not the direction we were heading.

Joshua her son seems to have things on his mind which Grace intends to tackle. Not sure what that's about, but I'm there for her and him regardless. Hoping that it's nothing to do with the two of us though, as Josh is aware of my condition. I do feel that we are heading in the direction of co-habiting it's as clear as daylight shines every day.

Her recent hint at applying for a job near where I reside was a clue in that direction. I do feel that I have found the right woman for me at long last, one whom I am very comfortable with and care about. Just wish I didn't have this disease, it just makes future planning extremely hard, more so as I am a realist.

9 May 2012

09:00 hours abiraterone tablets taken as described. 10:30 hours additional tablets taken as instructed. Attended doctor's surgery in the afternoon, needed to urgently pick up my Macmillan grant form which had been signed by my doctor.

Spent most of the day at my desk working without taking a break, it took a toll on my back and a little pain started which clearly was compounded, with me sitting at a table in my bedroom as opposed to lounge thus causing cramps to set in.

When will I learn about extending my legs under the table and sitting upright, correctly especially in my condition? The amount of times Grace has told me to do this as well as my doctors, sometimes I am so hard-headed or forgetful and do more harm than good to myself. Well early night as I felt extremely tired and have a heck of a day tomorrow.

As I reflect my mind pours on what my GP had suggested that I "think short term rather than long term" as regards to life expectancy. I'll never forget those words, nor a witness to them my brother who sat in with me at that particular appointment.

But here I was showing a miraculous comeback, those words being those of my hospital registrar doctor.

13 May 2012

09:00 hours abiraterone tablets taken as prescribed. 10:00 hours additional tablets taken as instructed. Nice lazy Sunday morning was had it was almost like the old days Grace's face was smiling and beaming and full of the love she has for me. She was a lady in full bloom and all because of me, and that made me feel loved and lovable. Funnily enough over the last two days I had no real time to think about my cancer pain or associated pains.

14 May 2012

08:00 hours abiraterone tablets taken as prescribed. Made contact with Hospital orthopaedic department to confirm appointment time which was given as 10:00 hours. At 09:00 hours additional tablets taken as instructed.

Arrived at the hospital at 10:20 hours, a little late filled in hospital form reference pre-op planning. The Stampede trials nurse came to see me to rearrange Wednesday's visit to Thursday 17th of May at 09:00 hours for blood pressure and bloods. At 12:20 hours I was seen by the surgeon who would be carrying out the operation. After a brief consultation clearance was given by him for the operation which would be around three to four weeks time under general anaesthesia, as an in-patient with a 48 hour recovery period after the operation.
I was quite surprised at the quickness of the intended operation. He is hoping that the pain will subside after this operation. Need to talk to doctor reference a lump that has come up in my throat since being discharged from hospital. In general, feeling not so stressed, not sure why this is as not much has changed in relation to my business affairs, maybe it's because I'm not concentrating on it so much.

15 May 2012

09:00 hours abiraterone tablets taken as prescribed. 11:00 hours additional tablets taken as instructed. After a tearful episode late last night I am feeling better. Don't know why I really cried, but Grace called me at the same time as I went into my tearful episode. Coincidental or angelic duties, I do wonder sometimes at the coincidences that occur between us.

Actually, I was at the time watching a movie on TV with Samuel L. Jackson "A Time to kill" and the scene at the time was where his daughter is assaulted.

Also something else was going on around me either a thought or something must have been there that pushed me to cry. MST taken 2 x 20 mg. My thought for today revolved around the fact that one of life's greatest tragedies is not to be loved. But I am and by many and this has kept me going regardless, but for those that aren't I really feel for you.

Today I reflected on my painful journey to date and realise that the human body is such a complex unit. There were many times when I came close to reaching the heights of pain tolerance level both mentally and physically. At age 54, I am still able to withstand an awful amount of pain way beyond that of a needle prick.

Luckily for me having kept reasonably fit my heart and mind were able to withstand much, but I wondered at times where my breaking point was and how close had I reached it on those occasions. I suppose dangerously close though.

17 May 2012

I awoke this morning at 01:30 hours and remained awake until 05:00 hours. Found that I was feeling very apprehensive in regard to my forthcoming operation which is geared for one week from today. Without a doubt my main concern was the fact that I would need to have a general anaesthetic, something I am not in favour of, or ever undergone. 07:00 hours abiraterone tablets taken as instructed. I have an appointment today with my oncologist as regards general update and well-being. 09:00 hours arrived at clinic A at local hospital. Weight taken given as 122.6kg blood pressure taken given as 165/79.

We discussed operation details for next week and to my amazement and joy she decided, that it would be in my best interests to cancel for now, the operation. She based this on the fact that my new PSA reading was now 123 which suggested a continued decline. Furthermore, she wanted to see the abiraterone tablets given more time to work on me.

Thus a delay of four weeks was proposed which would then take my participation in the stampede drug trials programme for three months. Should the pain not subside at the next consultation, then the option of the operation would be revisited.

There was also a suggestion that because I was going to have the operation, that this could be referred to the stampede drug trials committee, which worried her immensely in that they may see the pain issue as a failure of the abiraterone medication and hormone injection and with the results to date I was inclined to believe her and side with her recommendation and advice.

She further commented that she felt that my spine was not in a critical state and allowing the tablets and injection to continue to work would be far more advantageous to me. Now that the operation was cancelled it meant that all radiotherapy treatment would be placed on hold also. I agreed and the operation was officially cancelled, the sun could not have shone brighter than my facial expression at this decision.

Clearly now I understand why I was so uncomfortable earlier this morning and days past and I'm glad I stuck to my guns. I was advised that should I require Oramorph in future that the minimum dosage to be taken should be 5mg. I discussed about my enlarged throat, which she examined and informed me that this was more than likely lymph nodes caused through some sort of infection.

I can only say that I only developed this just after being discharged from hospital. I'm quite sure this was picked up on the ward as one patient was constantly coughing all over ward, that I'm sure is where I picked this up from.

I was advised that I should keep an eye on this to see if it enlarges further. Decided to shop in central London and buy Grace a well-deserved gift, an item that she showed me last Saturday whilst we were shopping in Covent Garden. She was reluctant to buy this clutch bag as she deemed it as being far too expensive. As far as I was concerned, she was worth it and I went to the shop "Hobbs" and purchased it.

I still have had a few surprises for her yet, smile. I have to say I'm in a good place mentally right now. Finances have cleared somewhat to the point of almost stress-free.

My personal love life seems to be on track, however, with some reservations in my mind. No longer do I feel that I am that cold mechanical human being. My children are and will always be the centre of my existence, but Grace has become a lady whom I have fallen in love with dearly and an integral part of the family and my existence. The ubiquitous hot flushes are really becoming a regular thing along with a very warm to hot feeling in my lower back area.

18 May 2012

09:00 hours abiraterone tablets taken as prescribed. 10:30 hours additional tablets taken as instructed. Feeling fairly good today so far, no real pains to complain about. Consciously keeping an eye on the lymph node in my throat. 14:00 hours Shopping with kids today and what a day this turned out to be. I decide to treat two of my daughters Lajade and Sam to a buy whatever you want day and they took that as a literal. Oxford Street in central London was descended upon by two teenagers and their father in tow and his wallet truly felt their wrath.

My finances took a boost this week and I found the stress had eased considerably, physically and mentally I was in a very good place which impacted on me physically also. After four hours of shopping my body felt the impact, especially in my lower back area but it was pleasurable to see my daughter's smiles, grins and poses as they were allowed to purchase whatever they wanted. This made me so happy as it had been a while since we were able to do something like this including lunch.

A perfect day was had. For another day my cancer concerns were forgotten and a smile returned to my face unlike any other day in recent times. Returned home at around 19:00 hours. Fortunately for me my eldest daughter Celena was able to pick me up from the tube station and drop me home. This was a blessing as the tiredness was evident upon me reaching home, by 20:30 hours I was in bed. It has to be said that fathers and their daughters do have special relationships.

Without a doubt the love in my two daughters eyes today was just more than Daddy buying them items of their hearts desire, but quality time was also had especially under the circumstances that prevail.

19 May 2012

09:00 hours abiraterone tablets taken as prescribed. 10:00 hours additional tablets taken as instructed. Out again shopping today with my eldest daughter Celena, today is her turn to be treated like her sisters the day before. Actually today was not so hectic as she knows what she wants, so back to Oxford Street again but to a limited area in fact a hundred meters from Oxford Street tube station just great though. It cost me more it was still worth it again to see how appreciative she was as she knew what she wanted and didn't want, but then at the age of 31 years she should do.
Lunch was at a Thai restaurant in south London around 16:00 hours. Returned home around 18:30 hours rested for about forty five minutes then it was football on TV my team Chelsea versus Bayer Munich. I

have been an avid supporter of Chelsea since 1967 the European cup was the trophy that eluded us and the game was just great and they won. I felt great and real happy that the team I supported were champions of Europe and the end of the match as this made me feel like a champion also. Kids kept testing me as to how happy they were with all the items that they had purchased over the last few days and wanted to thank me again. The smile remains on my face to this day. Well off to bed yet another day ahead tomorrow.

20 May 2012

09:00 hours abiraterone tablets taken as prescribed. 10:00 hours additional tablets taken as instructed. Grace arrived at 11:00 hours and off we went shopping to Costco, Tesco, and PC World. This was it for me my body was totally knackered though mentally I was okay but the fatigue is very much what I am suffering from. I am forgetting that I am not superman or super fit in any way, shape or form. But I was able to treat Grace for a nice gift as well as pay my way again after a few hard financial months of being very low, to no finances at all. She commented that over the past few days I was looking at ease and not so stressed out, I must say I have to agree. She loved her gift the clutch bag from Hobbs in Covent Garden.

21 May 2012

09:00 hours abiraterone tablets taken as prescribed. 10:30 hours additional tablets taken as instructed. My son and his girlfriend are in London today en-route to Gatwick airport so lunch and a nice chat are on the books. I am in a real happy mood as I've not seen him for a few months due to his professional football career and him residing in the Midlands.

We met at 13:00 hours and had a good time and chat. Met his girlfriend for the first time nice girl, but I personally don't think she's for him though, just a sixth sense, I guess, they are off to the Dominican Republic for seven days. Real good seeing my son as I just don't get to see enough of him, but I am so proud of him and all that he has achieved to date at the age twenty years. He left school with nine GCSE qualifications, but wanted a career in football, having come up through the Coventry city football academy scheme since the age of ten. He made it through the academy and was only one of three offered a professional contract upon reaching eighteen years.

My son will go far, mark my words and I hope I live long enough to witness his future success. Made contact with specialist cancer travel insurance companies. Insure blue Company only provides single trip no multiannual trips.

Contacted Age UK travel informed me that persons suffering with cancer for less than six months will usually have their applications declined. Further applications attempted for annual multi-trips were declined based on live activity whilst on stampede drug trial programme. Referred to another company free spirit, but still no success.

22 May 2012

Woke early around 04:00 hours with heavy sweating and hot flushes this is becoming very much the standard practice for me and my pillow upon waking each morning. This hormone treatment is definitely an emotional roller coaster; it screws with your head as well as your hormones. The symptoms are much like those experienced by women when they go through the change. Now I know how they really feel I can but empathise. 09:00 hours abiraterone tablets taken as prescribed. 10:00 hours additional tablets taken as instructed. Attended a major exhibition in London "ITEC" Stayed for about three hours before departing home, overall with travel and exhibition attendance seven hours was what it took. Mentally, I feel good, but physically totally exhausted; especially as the weather was exceptionally warm today in fact 75°C.

I found that I sweated a great deal more than usual. Luckily I carried a handkerchief with me, but this was drenched by the time I got home. Trousers I was wearing usually would be worn without the belt, however today I had to pull them up whilst in public, says much about my weight loss. Still find it hard to talk about my cancer to people who are just finding out about it, especially when you know they are looking at you with concern and trying to read you physically. I am very perceptive as to what is going on around me and appreciate what most people are trying to do, but, it does not make it any easier or better for me to deal with. Had a heart-to-heart talk with Grace tonight as regards me and my attitude to our predicament and the fact that I may be around for a long or not so long period of time. She does not like to hear when I talk like this even though she realises that I am a realist.

I see the hurt in her eyes when this discussion happens. She seems though now to be more amenable to my views on this now and allows me to rant about. The other night whilst in bed we talked and she told me she would marry me tomorrow if she could. What's stopping that from being a reality is clearly my reluctance to do so as I feel it would not be proper or correct at this stage of the treatment for us to wed. It's still early days in my cancer battle and she understands this, but I do hear and appreciate the sentimental proposal.

Josh, her son and I seem to be getting on much better these last few months. Not that we had any bad words or ill feeling previously it just seems like a better atmosphere all around exists. I know Grace views this as very important and it means so much to her. I am so happy about this as this young man I treat and care for as if he were my own blood son. Really starting to take care of my body, from a health perspective and am eating and drinking better than before.

23 May 2012

Woke early again at 04:30 hours still experiencing sweating along with hot flushes. I have noticed and felt a heat rush in my chest upwards to my head and a sickly feeling in my stomach during this rush which does not last for more than twenty to twenty five minutes. 08:00 hours abiraterone tablets taken as prescribed.

Busy day today I have to attend a luncheon function at the House of Lords, hosted by a member of the house.

My work takes me into different circles currently my company is in the process of organising a special counterterrorism conference to be held in the Caribbean later this year. This would focus on Platinum Command and Control as regards Policing, Military and Civilian events.

In attendance at this function were a number of business associates and overseas government colleagues. The luncheon event was excellent, and a good day was had by all in attendance.

One of the highlights of the day was a tour of the House of Lords and parts of the House of Commons. Parliament is steeped in history and we found it totally exciting and thrilling and actually got a buzz from it all. The days' event was most definitely tiring combined with sweating, hot flushes and I almost got to the point of passing out, though I did not tell anyone until after we had left the House of Lords. Obviously a suit and tie were the occasion and these did not help me to keep cool, especially due to the exceptional weather today which exceeded 25°C.

I have to say without a doubt this particular Lord was a most humble, articulate, intelligent and jovial man, not what I expected from a person of such title to be perfectly honest. In the esteemed company that I sat with and the distinguished visual surroundings, I learned an awful amount today. I must say Grace looked exceptionally beautiful and I felt proud to have her on my arm and accompanying me to such an historical and exquisite place. She enjoyed the day and the whole proceedings added a marvellous touch to our relationship a sense of real appreciation of one another was felt.

Felt a little unwell towards the latter part of the day and just put this down to the sweating, hot flushes, fatigue and the excessive heat due to wearing a suit and tie. How I did not faint will remain one of life's mysteries. Early to bed on our return at 20:30 hours to be precise. My body just closed down immediately once we arrived home. Weather is predicted to be very sunny over the week and I need to remember to drink plenty of water.

24 May 2012

Woke around 04:00 hours found that I was extremely physically wet and very uncomfortable and irritable for about thirty minutes whilst I lay there. Things eventually calmed down and I managed to sleep for a few hours further. 09:00 hours abiraterone tablets taken as prescribed. 10:00 hours additional tablets taken as instructed. Contacted an old friend of mine and informed him of my condition. He was totally stunned by the news and I could hear it in his voice and his genuine concern for my welfare. He told me about a friend that got cancer twice and on one occasion diagnosed as terminal and actually got paid out by the insurance company, but survived and cleared himself of cancer and remains alive today.

All in the mind Pete says and I do agree without a doubt. Today I must say Grace is a great part of that desire and willingness to survive and spend my remaining years with her in whatever loving manner befits us, obviously my children are the other part of that desire to stay alive. Grace and I went to a sauna tonight as we both needed it even though today's temperatures were in excess of 80°C. We still ventured to the sauna as it offered a different set of therapeutic values.

It was great, especially for Grace, who had come home tonight in a real state after a bad day at work. In fact, very close to tears she was as she recounted her last few days whilst I listened sympathetically. It was at this point that I knew she needed a pick me up in the form of a sauna.

Well 22:00 hours we arrived and departed at 23:40 hours somewhat unusually short but nonetheless worthwhile I usually stay longer, but this was her first time so maybe next time.

I can only say that she was a new person after the sauna though somewhat facially drained of colour her mood and temperament were evident. I myself felt that with all that had been going on in my life as well as hers she had reached saturation point. The sauna had brought her back.

25 May 2012

Woke at 07:30 hours both Grace and I. She is working from home today and what a different lady she seems today. Her face has a glow to it and she stated she felt totally re-energised and ready to go again.

Must say I felt a great sense of satisfaction in seeing the Grace I know back in almost full stride. As I sit here at 08:10 hours I am dripping with sweat all over my bed sheets it's going to be a scorcher again today without a doubt.

Must make sure I drink more water than juices. Last night once again Grace and I had one of our heart-to-heart talks with reference to solidifying our relationship that being marriage as she does not have any issues with my prognosis. However, I do and I feel we should wait a bit longer before committing. It's not that I don't want to settle with her it's just that I would want to feel in my mind that it was for a longer period of time and not based on my GP's theory of short-term. I am quite clear in my mind what I want for both myself and Grace and our family. I know that after almost 4 months, since being diagnosed and what I've gone through to date that the battle has not yet started. Grace told me something last night that made me feel confident that I can beat this disease.

She said whilst observing me in A&E that my desire and will to live were evident and my words whilst under duress "This is not going to get me" were examples of that positive attitude. I have felt very alone a lot during the past few weeks though so many people have shown an interest in my welfare, I just still feel alone in my fight at times and no one really cares other than my immediate family. I suppose as I reflect, I am seeing that I have a very needy disposition emerging which I need to get a handle on before too long.

I still have not done my will as yet and need to get this done urgently; I don't understand why I'm dilly dallying about this important matter. 09:00 hours abiraterone tablets taken as prescribed. 10:00 hours additional tablets taken as instructed. My back feels rested and not so painful to me. I'm returning home to Mitcham today, Grace will drive me over as she always does. Got a little surprise for her today been planning this for a while.

Weather again today was very hot though I was not sweating and feeling my usual hot flushes. Gave Grace a very nice surprise as we drove towards my home, I re-directed her to the high street shops - I have for weeks seen a black dress that I felt was just made for her so we went and bought the dress though not the one I exactly or really liked as her size was not available, so she choose another one that she adored and it showed on her face without a doubt.

She looked $1 million in this dress today little does she know there is a bigger surprise yet to come. She deserves it without a doubt and it's my little way of saying thanks again. I suppose a simple thank you would suffice for many but, not for my Grace as in my mind, she is an exceptional kind human being without a doubt.

Grace is a lovely lady and I do love her dearly, but during lunch today we both decided that we had to really lay our feelings down as to how we saw our relationship and my sickness. We agreed that we needed to think matters out seriously and plan carefully our future. I have to say as I have many times that without her attentiveness, and love that things would have most definitely been different and possibly in a negative way.

I checked again online this evening as to insurance for a cancer patient and was not surprised that the statement declining persons while still receiving treatment for cancer and the fact that you could still be declined for up to four to five years after remission came back. This clearly impacted on our plans to buy a home together, but as one door shuts I say another will open, we are determined to find a way to be together and I have to say I feel alive again, in that someone is taking an interest in me making me feel that we do have a future together after all.

26 May 2012

09:00 hours abiraterone tablets taken as prescribed. 10:00 hours additional tablets taken as instructed. A glorious day today, it's already in the 80's and it's only 10:00 hours.

Today is exactly four months to the day since I was diagnosed with advanced metastatic prostate cancer. Can't say I feel any different about it other than my PSA levels have come down from just over 501 to 123 since then. Mentally, I still feel in turmoil as its early days yet and the effect on my life has been horrendously up heaving, but I fight on.

Some people in my life say cancer is a mind thing, well let me tell you, it's both mind and physical and one has to be strong to withstand the onslaught that you are put through.

Over the months I have gone through the deep thought process of revaluating who my true friends are and what is the true meaning of LOVE of another human being. This has allowed me to understand that my relationship with my partner was truly a scrutiny of love. I have also understood the reality and depth of the trials programme medically.

The uncertainties and disorganisation that surrounds this very new programme is amazing, and I have complied with all requested off me throughout and more. I am clearly piggy in the middle in this game of chess and chance, but what held me together were my constant conversations with god. He showed me the way and to fear nothing placed before me. On a daily basis between 09:00 hours and 18:30 hours, I really had no other real human companion or contact to converse with, hence my daily life was really a lonely one.

I have withstood the pain, the tears, the sense of loss of emotional feelings and my manliness, which in itself I can tell you is as hard as fighting the cancer itself. In defining manliness the best description that I can find to describe the word is "being the best man you can be". So often I have questioned myself, was I being the best man to my partner? Our sex life was non-existent, with all the medication taken could I ever have an orgasm again. I questioned constantly how my partner felt about the situation, I personally needed answers as what affected me, affected her. So I raised the question and the answer I got back made me have to really re-think what relationships are all about. In her words "She abstained from intimacy for a number of years, so it was not a real issue to her". Well knock me down with a feather when I heard that, here I was concerned about a very personal and private matter after only five months. All I could say was point taken and lesson learnt I thought to myself.

The loss financially to my business and the stressful effect that this has had on me has impacted greatly on my mind and body. The suffering is beyond a doubt a symbol of the struggle encountered and I have withstood all, though at times it was touch and go. Let's see what the next few months bring, maybe I'll be one of the fortunate ones and survive to tell my story.

27 May 2012

09:00 hours abiraterone tablets taken as prescribed. 10:00 hours additional tablets taken as instructed. Today's weather was extremely hot combined with hot flushes I found it harder to function fully. My mid back area was still causing me pain and discomfort. Last night a pain took a hold of me, in the mid back area that caused me to raise and arch my back once again. For a few minutes the pain was mild to severe then it just eased away, but on hand close by I had the Oramorph break through medication just in case.

Tonight I had dinner at my daughters Celena's home and we had a father daughter talk about my partner Grace and our intended future life, relationship and our plans for the future which she seemed to warm to. This made me feel so glad that my eldest daughter approves or at the very least seemed to approve. Always a sticky area to try and talk about but today went without hitch. I know my daughters well enough and this made my whole day, month, and year. Sent Grace a text about it all but joked slightly, she was glad in the end that the outcome was positive and that we could move on, not that everything would have stopped there and then. Mentally, I am in a very good place indeed. 23:30 hours last set of tablets taken as per instructions.

28 May 2012

09:00 hours abiraterone tablets taken as prescribed. 10:00 hours additional tablets taken as instructed. Another hot day combined with the occasional hot flushes caused me to feel overheated. Other than that I felt good. Busy day out on the road achieved a number of things. Due to the excessive heat felt tired earlier than usual. Fell asleep early evening and woke up feeling very hot at 23:30 hours, just in time to take my night-time medication. Took my temperature reading which was 36.5 which is actually normal. Other than that, feel okay, no real pains to complain about at this moment in time.

29 May 2012

08:00 hours abiraterone tablets taken as prescribed. 09:00 hours additional tablets taken as instructed. Still very hot weather we are experiencing but I felt good today. Hospital appointment today at 11:00 hours. Bloods taken and blood pressure also taken reading

150/91 with a pulse of 76. Discussed at length re-supply of drugs on a long-term basis. The trials nurse arranged total re-supply that allowed me to pick up MST, Prednisolone and Omeprazole tablets supply at the hospital pharmacy.

Also confirmed a new consultant appointment, which is arranged for 17th July. I do feel however that they need to get their act together in regards to sorting out my appointments in general as this makes me feel nervy and affects my lifestyle. Received a telephone call from a doctor at the Royal Marsden hospital, reference radiotherapy treatment as a result of a letter request from my local hospital. I was under the impression that this had been cancelled like the operation, I requested they confirm this with my local hospital oncology team.

As the weather was not so hot today my energy levels were good and I did not feel sapped of energy nor experiencing any hot flushes. Contacted Macmillan support with regards to my recent application submitted for new clothing as I had not heard anything to date. Support worker confirmed that that application had been signed off and approved and I should hear something within the next ten days. Today I learnt something new "the best things in THIS LIFE are always hidden. You have to be a seeker to find what is good."

30 May 2012

Woke up early with sweating issues, I was soaked from head to chest. At this moment in time this is becoming the norm and is very uncomfortable. My pillow and bed sheets are soaked from my bodily perspiration, especially my pillow which is actually soaked all the way through. My son arrived back in the UK today from holiday with his girlfriend; glad that he's back safe and sound can't stop worrying about my children, no matter where they are. I'm not an over compulsive worrier, but the world we live in now, differs greatly from my days and is far more dangerous and I suppose that's what concerns me most. 09:00 hours abiraterone tablets taken as prescribed. 10:15 hours additional tablets taken as instructed.

Met up with my son at Victoria Station at 11:00 hours and spent the day with him before he departed back to the Midlands where he resides.

His girlfriend had to go to an embassy in London to get a visa for travel in July. Therefore, it was one on one, quality time between father and son. To be totally honest, it has been a while since my son and I have had time to spend together due to his football career, but today I was a very happy, happy father. My boy has made me so proud and I know that I continue to say this, but I am extremely proud of my son. As each day passes I wonder to myself how was I so blessed with a son such as him, to this date he has never been in trouble with the police, nor found himself in bad company and is always courteous and polite to all that meet him. I know some of this was to do with his upbringing, but peer pressure is something we parents can lose a child behaviour and future to, but we never did.

We talked at length about the number of things, including him purchasing his first home, which apparently "exchange of keys" is set for the 31/5/12, wow, what a special occasion for him again I'm so proud of this landmark in his life. We talked about his football future and I gave him my advice, which seemed to coincide with his general thoughts and viewpoints. We travelled on the underground rail system and sat side-by-side and for the first time I realised how physically large he was from a chest and shoulder point of view. Also how strong he was as I nudged him I felt the strength of a young powerful man, he is going be a giant in his later years as he is only 20 years now and stands at six-foot one already.

A young man that you would call a gentle giant in the making. For me, today was an excellent day and allowed me again to be treated to a rare moment of being able to forget my woes, worries, and pains.

We also discussed my current medical situation and I brought him up to date with current treatments and results.

The day went so fast and we had to part, for me that was the tearful moment unknown to him, but he was hoping to be back in London for a planned family get-together which was pencilled in for the Monday, June 4th, so I was glad to hear that though it might not happen nonetheless glad to hear it.

Managed to contact local hospital and obtain the latest PSA results taken on the 29th May, result given was 48 WOW, WOW, WOW elated was not the word but it will do for now it's all heading in the right direction. Shared the news with family, though, I still am in pain in my lower back area. It is my view that if the pain continues then the radiotherapy treatment is just round the corner.

With every lowering of my PSA results I am more determined to beat this dreadful cancer disease that has invaded my body and that of my family of the past. You are not going to win, oh no you don't, how dare you think you can beat me, after the fight that I have put up and still put up for my lovely adorable children and let's not forget my partner Grace and stepson Josh for without them maybe none of this would have been possible. Felt quite tired after such a busy day so retired just before 22:00 hours. Intend to take it easy for the rest of the week. Last of the day's tablets taken.

31 May 2012

Woke in the early hours with a severe pain to my left side, around the hip and thigh areas, which pulsated for about a few minutes or so. It faded out and I was able to sleep thereafter. 09:00 hours abiraterone tablets taken 10:00 hours additional tablets taken as instructed. Today I have become the following person, a possibilitarian. I have realised who I am and what I have gone through to date, I am not afraid of tomorrow for God is already there. Rested most of the day until early evening then went to Caribbean restaurant and had a fishmeal consisting of steamed fish with bammy. For those who do not know what Bammy is, it is a traditional Jamaican cassava flatbread descended from the simple flatbread. Tablets taken as usual, however later than usual, this did not seem to affect me, but just left an uncomfortable feeling in my stomach.

1 June 2012

I awoke early due to the sweating again as per the last few days. 09:00 hours abiraterone tablet taken as prescribed. 10:00 hours additional tablets taken as instructed. Physically felt good today, no real pain to complain about just aches but that's the usual. Mentally felt in a place of solitude, but all alone. Excessive sweating poured out of my body again as per previous days.

As it is the weekend Grace is picking me up later, so I'm looking forward to that in fact I am quite apprehensive to be honest. Spoke to a friend Peter and had a lengthy conversation with him as there seems to be a misunderstanding going around about my illness, as does happen when too many people know, along the way one can expect variations or distortions of the truth I suppose. Grace and I had another of our heart-to-heart talks tonight and I laid down some hard truths for her to grasp.

I know she tends not to want to think about the possibility of my demise. So I told her about a dream I recently had about my funeral and that she was there as well as Josh her son and that she fainted and Josh caught her just in time. They do say one does not dream straight, but nonetheless I told her.

Many tears were shed as she repeated "I don't know what I'm going to do without you should you die," she has a tendency to keep her back to me when she utters words of distraught and not let me see her tears. Today I saw them; today I saw how in love with me she is. Today I decided to clear the air in that I wanted her to know that I wish her happiness now and also long after, and that she should not allow herself to pine for me too long. We both agreed that should our relationship be able to last fifteen to twenty years at our ages now, then why would we really want anyone else in our life after saying ages sixty five to seventy years. But for now I'll take all the quality time that I can get for us to spend.

Spoke with my daughter Celena for thirty minutes today as she is attending a family function on her mother's side of the family. She is quite unhappy about attending as she and her mother do not see eye to eye nor really communicate. It was very evident at this time of the morning to hear how she felt and all I could do or say was to offer words of comfort and fatherly advice.

Celena's childhood years were in my care, so she only knew me as her mother and father and it has always, been a battle for her, to recognise her mother as a mother. It hurts my heart to see her in this anguish, because deep down I know she yearns for her mother's love, which her mother just can't seem to give her.

Just one word from her mother showing affection and speaking it would make her day. I have found that I am best placed to stay to one side in this situation, however, as I go through my illness I find that I am coming to the opinion that I may have to at some stage intervene, not something I'm looking forward to having to do, but I hate to see my daughter in this place and undergoing this emotional distress that she has had to endure all these years.

As I told her a few months ago, make peace with your mother as I won't always be around but as she said in return, I know dad and that's what worries me, a tear rolled down my face with her response.

2 June 2012

09:00 hours abiraterone tablets taken as prescribed. 10:00 hours additional tablets taken as instructed. Sweating still causing me to have uneasy nights' my forehead and chest areas of my body are the main areas of the sweat concentration. Lower back is still causing me concern, stiff at times and painful. This evening attended a rock concert Emirates Stadium, the band Coldplay. Grace and a good friend of mine Peter Hillier came along. It was partly business as well as pleasure. It was very cold and as a cancer patient I felt the extremity of the cold; it just went through me like a hot knife through butter. Nonetheless a good night was had by all of us.

3 June 2012

Sweating made me wake early today along with a feeling of suffocation primarily coming from the throat area. 09:30 hours abiraterone tablets taken as prescribed. 10:30 hours additional tablets taken as per instructions. Felt very strange today I found myself in the place of confusion and non-communication with Grace. She would converse with me and I either did not reply, or when I did it did not make sense what I said, she said. Along with a general lack of energy to pull myself out of bed, I was not in a good place at all.

This was a first for me in all my years being mentally confused. The day got progressively better for me though. I decided that I would allow my partner Grace to participate in my symptom journal. I asked her if she would do so and she willingly accepted what follows now is an extract in her words written by myself today Sunday 3 June 2012. "One of the things that struck me this morning was how disorientated and grumpy you were. I had to ask you the same question several times to get an answer from you, which was very unusual.

I put this down to the very restless night that you had. After eating it seemed that the grogginess wore off and you were okay for the rest of the day. There was no uneasiness between us as the night before we had words between us over a misunderstanding, but we were back to our usual self thereafter.

You knew my friend was coming over for dinner (someone she had known for over 20 years and was dying to meet the man that had put life's smile back in her face) and I asked you the question, do you have an issue with this? To which you replied no I do not (evidently it's the small things that matter, where women are concerned).

She continues - though I was in the kitchen preparing Sunday dinner most of the time, I intermittently would come out to see how you were. I recall asking you nearer the time of the arrival of my friend if you were going to change your clothes and spruce yourself up which you complied to.

I felt a sense of comfort during and after dinner and in my mind hoped that this was reflective, in your mind also as I was in a very happy place. You were relaxed and at ease and that was all that I cared about. I felt really happy, proud and pleased to spend the day with you.

You were not afraid to express your feelings for me in front of my friend and you still were your playful self, cuddling and kissing me and showing your care and affection for me. What really made me feel happy was that after dinner, my friend Marcia offered to clear the table, but you said no and both you and I cleared the table as if we were both entertaining a guest in our own home. At this moment in time a text message comes from her friend Marcia, who had left to go home stating that Alfred is a diamond geezer.

I noted that during the day that there were no real signs of pain or wincing things which are the normal that I observe.

I was so glad that it was a long holiday weekend Queen's Jubilee and that you did not have to leave to go home as would be the usual on a Sunday after dinner or sometimes earlier. I don't really have much more to add other than I really feel lucky to have you in my life". As I dictate I can see the tears of happiness and love in her eyes with a certain twinkle that she gives off like a satisfied feline when content.

4 June 2012

09:30 hours abiraterone tablets taken as prescribed. 11:00 hours additional tablets taken as instructed. Today was a bank holiday,

Grace and I treated it as a day of rest though we were due at a family gathering on my side of the family at 17:00 hours in South London. I felt fairly okay throughout the day, though; I am urinating far more than usual need to check my sugar levels.

No real pains to complain about at present. Received a phone call at 14:00 hours, which infuriated me. My daughter Kira and son Nathan from Birmingham were on their way to London, but family accommodation for them had not being fully arranged. I was outraged as I thought the family had sorted this out, clearly not. I found myself so stressed out trying to sort it out at such short notice.

This was not happening and I called the family meal off, which put me in a foul mood and I became tearful as I had to inform them both that it was off due to no accommodation being arranged by the family and I was not happy to have them stay today on a sofa. All this means is that I need to make sure I get my act together and buy a new home that would sort that issue from happening again like how it used to be. Decided to go to bed early as I was in a foul mood.

5 June 2012

09:30 hours abiraterone tablets taken as prescribed. 10:30 hours additional tablets taken as instructed. Another bank holiday spent very quietly with Grace. We decided to sort out a few personal matters and follow up on our recent discussions. We decided to create an online banking flexi account and filled out a list of questions.

Decided to look at the City & Guilds training course Teacher training certificate. Few other things sorted out and it felt good that Grace and I sat down and did it together. Made me feel human as did the sexual arousal that I seem to have coming back in me for her as one of the side effects of the medication is loss of sexual libido.

Today for the first time in many months I found myself sexually aroused and erect whilst lying in bed with her. My desire to make love to her was forthcoming, though it did not happen there and then, it still meant that a massive part of my life was coming back which I could share with her.

My sexual manliness may be gradually coming back but, I am very concerned that this could be short-term and that my next three monthly injections, which are due within the next few weeks will send everything backwards. It's an awful thing when your sexual prowess ceases and you are unable to be a real man, especially as you have been used to this as a certain way of life. I found myself withdrawing from not only my family, but my partner as I began to notice the change in my body and my self-image. Clearly I needed time to adjust to the way I felt about myself and how I looked to others. This is why I knew how special our relationship was under the varying circumstances.

6 June 2012

09:00 hours abiraterone tablets taken as described. 10:00 hours additional tablets taken as instructed. Felt very hot due to hot flushes mainly in my head and chest area. My daughter Kira's 24th birthday today and I rang her and wished her well and the best as always, she was glad to hear my voice and I am so happy being alive to wish her happy birthday. Contacted GP for appointment reference lymph-node on the right side of throat, appointment given as Thursday 14th at 09:00 hours.

The sweating is really becoming frequent and making me uncomfortable. A few red pimples similar to rashes are apparent in the chest area of my body. No major pains in other parts of my body. Still felt hotter than usual. Decided to make contact with on-call doctor and oncology department.

Called them at 22:00 hours and informed them of the things I was going through doctor advised that these could be attributed to side effects of the trial programme drugs.

General advice was to hold off until next oncology visit which was June 20th and if still a problem then to discuss it there and then with the consultant. I must say that Grace has seen the increase in these conditions and it worries her as much as me. The weather today is quite mild yet I still sweat like a pig and shiver too. Early night tonight let's see what tomorrow brings.

7 June 2012

09:00 hours abiraterone tablets taken as described. 10:00 hours additional tablets taken as instructed. Still profusely sweating, sweat pouring off my face. Stayed at home today as the sweating made me feel very uncomfortable as well as I am not feeling physically myself, just feel stiff and non-flexible. Felt that I needed to get back into the gym like I used too if and when I felt that way.

Kids seem very quiet these last few days I miss hearing from them maybe Celena thinks I'm mad with her reference Nathan and Kira but I'm not. Getting ready now to get back to Mitcham being here at Grace's just over one week now. Reflected back today on the day each of my children were born. My existence on this earth was about them, they gave me the inspiration to do better in this world they saved my life then and they never really knew.

You see the path I was on then was the path of total destruction and I owe them my life, hence my reason and desire to achieve in life so that they do not have to ever to go down my previous path. I love them all dearly without them I have nothing and am nothing. Maybe one day they will all understand their father, maybe one day they will all have the chance to read an autobiography of my life.

Once again my thoughts rest on one of my encouraging choice of words "Possibilitarian". No matter how dark things seemed to be or actually were, when faced with a problem that was created from circumstances beyond my control I continued to raise my sights to see the possibilities ahead I always saw them, for they were always there.

It's now just over six months since I was diagnosed with this illness, during which fear and panic had set in, because I had this terrible illness. Did I know what my fate was, no I did not, but in asking myself this question does anyone ever know what there's.

Over the past months the continuous prodding, blood tests and medical checks have left me feeling jaded and low in esteem. The moments of feeling well, strong and healthy were few and far between and on those occasions I could mistakenly think that I was cancer free.

Clearly on-going tests are to be a way of life for me with regards to this advance prostate cancer and accepting this is not easy at all. There exists in our family a cancer history and the susceptibility to both breast cancer and prostate gene have some resonance with each other as my mother, aunt, uncle and three cousins all died from either breast or prostate related cancer issues. Just when you think it can't get any worse it does. In the treatment of my cancer the prostap hormone injection was by far the worst aspect of this treatment I suppose anything that induces a sort of castration of manhood would do.

8 June 2012

09:00 hours abiraterone tablets taken as prescribed. 10:00 hours additional tablets taken as per instructions. Still sweated a lot actually it dripped from off of me. Cleary it seemed to be the hot flush side-effects of the cancer treatment hormone injection that caused this. Went shopping in central London today and had a good walk out and about. Weather was coldish which did not help matters, very windy in fact. Received a telephone call from a client in the United States reference an assignment in Brazil São Paulo for the July/August months. Need to look into this properly and see if I can be ready for then.

9 June 2012

Woke early again drenched due to sweats. Shared a joke with Grace in that we both are suffering from the issue of hot flushes. Now I know how women feel when they go through that moment. I asked myself what a way to understand what a woman goes through on a regular basis by suffering with them. I tell you it's horrendous, the feeling of your energy been sapped from your body as well as the damp body/clothing feeling, sometimes the clothing actually clung to the body. 09:00 hours abiraterone tablets taken as described. 10:00 hours additional tablets taken as per instructions.

Today I felt very moody and needy and found myself crying towards the early part of the evening in front of Grace, fortunately she understood and consoled me, but I just felt so vulnerable when this happened, very vulnerable indeed.

10 June 2012

09:00 hours abiraterone tablets taken as prescribed. 10:00 hours additional tablets taken as per instructions. Sweats are still occurring, felt low and needy again, and again tearful which resulted in quite a few tearful moments again during the day. Once again Grace was there for me though I felt for her, in that she does not know what she can do for me other than try to console me when it occurs.

It's a funny feeling isn't it that I feel the same when she has the same feelings, but I can't do anything for her neither, but I do understand.

We decided to have Sunday lunch out today, just felt that I needed to get out more and be among people. Grace was excellent company, though she became tearful as she dropped me home later.

Parting is getting harder between us both as we spend more time together. Grace stated that sometime soon we need to have a one-to-one as regards parts of her life unknown to me that she would like to share.

I have always felt that there was more and time would be the revealer as regards this aspect. We are becoming closer and closer and without a doubt lifelong partners I feel it in my blood.

11 June 2012

09:00 hours abiraterone tablets taken as prescribed. 11:00 hours additional tablets taken as instructed. I'm now back home after being away for another week at Grace's. Getting used to not being around her again is painful, especially when I have to put up with a bed that is so low and I find it difficult to get up out of. My chairs are uncomfortable and cause me some pain after sitting in them for long periods of time. Today I looked at myself in the mirror and thought I'm just so fed up with trying to look reasonably well for someone of my age and ailment. I shaved often and trimmed the grey areas, but there comes a point when you just say to hell with it just leave it alone. The sweating seems to be a day-to-day thing, though I felt just slightly warmish. I feel that I need time to myself to make some firm decisions with regards to what is ahead (I mean what I know is).

Received the cheque today from Macmillan Cancer support for £250 towards new clothes. It won't go far, but nonetheless it was still nice to receive this amount. The TV adverts that show far more regular than at any time before don't go half way to understanding how invaluable an organisation like this has become. I was thinking about the amount of tablets I take a day now to stay alive; it's 14 each day.

Abiraterone acetate tablets 250mg – Four tablets once daily on empty stomach. No food to be consumed for at least two hours before the dose and for at least 1 hour after the dose.

Omeprazole Gastro-resistant capsules 20mg – One to be taken twice a day.

Prednisolone tablets 5mg. - One tablet once a day with or just after food or a meal.

Morphine Sulphate controlled release tablets 10mg – Two to be taken twice a day Avoid alcohol – If sleepy do not drive/use machines

Ibuprofen Tablets 400mg – One to be taken three times day with or just after food or a meal.

Additionally, there is the Oramorph Oral Solution 10mg/5ml Morphine sulphate – For break through pain ONLY. This is only to be taken when the pain is severe between regular medication times.

It's so funny how in tune Grace has become with me, I stated earlier, I needed time to myself and I intended to take some sort of action which I knew would cause major upset. Within an hour of me writing and thinking what I wrote earlier, Grace telephoned twice, however, I ignored these calls and then she texted me, it read "Hi hubby just making sure all is ok unusual for you not to respond to me..G xxx" the second text read "I knew something was up today I could not shake off the feeling that all was not well with you and just got more anxious as the day went on". Clearly this stopped me from doing something which would have hurt her and others emotionally, but it's how I felt and I had to say how I felt. Appointment set for blood pressure and bloods on Thursday 14th June. Also appointment set for 10:30 hours with oncologist for Wednesday 20th of June at 15:00 hours. Well, let's see if my PSA level goes down into single figures that would really pick me up and I suppose everyone else. Made a real concerted effort today to eat healthily and cook freshly myself. Still felt the hot flushes in my head, body, and arms. The sweats are still very much apparent, but not as much as over the last few days. Still felt unclear what to do about my professional career and prospective work contracts forthcoming much to think about still.
12 June 2012

09:00 hours abiraterone tablets taken as prescribed. I forgot to take my tablets at 10:00 hours and only realised it at 21:45 hours so I just took steroids and MST plus Ibuprofen, and Omeprazole at 23:00 hours. Last night I forgot to take MST and Ibuprofen tablets at 23:00 hours, I need to ensure that I do not do this regularly to ensure continuity of response to medication. Today I felt very cold within my body and sweats came back with a clamminess about it. Need to arrange extra heater at home.

09:00 hours abiraterone tablets taken as described. 10:30 hours additional tablets taken as instructed. Attended doctor's surgery in the afternoon, needed to urgently pick up my Macmillan grant form which had been signed by my doctor. Spent most of the day at my desk working without taking a break, it took a toll on my back and a little pain started which clearly was compounded, with me sitting at a table in my bedroom as opposed to lounge thus causing cramps to set in.

When will I learn about extending my legs under the table and sitting upright correctly especially in my condition? The amount of times Grace has told me to do this as well as my doctors, sometimes I am so hard-headed or forgetful and do more harm than good to myself. Well early night as I felt extremely tired and have a heck of a day tomorrow.

As I reflect my mind reflects on what my GP had suggested that I "think short term rather than long term" as regards to life expectancy. I'll never forget those words, nor a witness to them my brother who sat in with me at that particular appointment.

But here I was showing a miraculous comeback, those words being those of my hospital registrar doctor.

13 June 2012

Woke early due to over sweating, pillow and quilt liner are very damp, could not go to sleep so laid and thought for a while before getting up and going online on my computer to surf and pass the time. Saw an article whilst online reference Peter Andre the artist, whose brother has liver and bladder cancer. It stated that it had spread. This dampened my spirits somewhat, especially the bit referring to the fact that his care treatment was under Royal Marsden Hospital cancer treatment hospital in the UK. Now I don't know his brother or him, so why was it so readily affecting me. Anyone that had cancer was readily affecting me it seemed.

I kept saying that I should not take notice of Internet features on cancer, but this one was very different in that it referred to the hospital that my dear mother underwent her treatment. I left an e-mail for Grace at 04:00 hours just referring to my loneliness as well as the article on Peter Andre's brother.

09:00 hours abiraterone tablets taken as prescribed. 10:00 hours additional tablets taken as instructed. Received a call from Grace at around 11:30 hours reference to email I sent earlier. She sensed my mood on the telephone, there is no hiding my feelings where she is concerned. I've made up my mind to relocate within the next four weeks as the care and attention and needs are just not at my fingertips. Looks like I will be moving in with Grace which was contrary to my recent discussions with her that I would reside south of the London as opposed to where she lived in North West London, Middlesex.

This is a temporary measure and one that I have made clear. But I'm very thankful for this as I really did not have many other options available, which would not compromise me. Started to clear out all papers by shredding as I want to limit clutter that I have. My brother Kelly came over and we had a chat about a couple of business contracts forthcoming in 2013 which would financially put me in a very good place.

As stated to him if I am healthy and obviously alive then I would consider these contracts. Feeling fairly well in myself other than the sweats, once again, my back is playing me up, but this is due to a bad chair that I am sitting on.

Decided I'd call a family meeting after my hospital appointment next week Wednesday, I needed to clear the air as I felt that I was losing the closeness of my family.

I felt as if there was a distance being created for one reason or another and it made me very sad. I need my children around me more than anything else in this world. Their happiness is my ultimate goal regardless of what is happening to me there is no replacement for me their father.

14 June 2012

08:00 hours abiraterone tablets taken as prescribed. 09:00 hours additional tablets taken as instructed. Today I have an appointment with my GP at the surgery to discuss the sweating and lump that has come up in my throat. He stated that MST will cause excessive sweating along with the steroids, which will increase the weight. He further stated that I need to drink much more water and I also needed to wear looser clothing to keep cool in hot weather along with open sandals instead of shoes or trainers with air mesh and no socks. He examined the lump in my throat and stated I should ask the specialist to do a biopsy on it. He personally had no idea of what it was.

To be honest, this GP has never filled me with confidence at all and I found myself asking other questions which received equally no proper medical answers. I just wanted to tell him to go to hell, but stopped short, as I knew this was almost the last time that he would be acting as my GP, as I was relocating would mean registering with a new GP Surgery. Attended hospital for my bloods and Blood Pressure appointment at 10:30 hours blood pressure reading 160/92 slightly high, bloods were also taken.

The good thing is that this was the last time I had to attend this clinic appointment as the 12 week period has now elapsed. From here on in it will be every six weeks for my consultation with the oncologist. The lump in my throat is worrying me a bit after the doctor stated that a biopsy should be carried out. I sent a text message out to kids requesting a family meeting so that I can really sort things out from a family perspective.

I failed to mention that when I woke this morning I did not have the sweats. I wore a heavy kind of jumper to bed last night and I hardly sweated, just don't understand it at all. Though this afternoon at 15:50 hours I sweated like a pig it was pouring off me.

Well, next week I have a consultation appointment with the oncology team and I have a list of questions ready for them.

Well, it's now confirmed I will be moving from where I currently reside to west London. I have mixed feelings about this, but I know it's on a temporary basis just hope the kids will understand that.

Started packing even though I am a month away from the actual move date, but I realise that I still cannot manage heavy items too well, so I will have to seek some assistance from male family members.

15 June 2012

09:00 hours abiraterone tablets taken as prescribed. 10:00 hours additional tablets taken as instructed. I spent most of the day shredding documents in anticipation of my move. It's amazing how much junk was amassed over the six years I had resided here.

Kind of happy though, as I can now see some sort of order and structure coming back into my business life. Bowel movements, returning. Clearly this week I've looked after myself better by eating and cooking the right things and though this evening I pigged out, an added treat of double cheeseburger and chips along with ice cream. Well, I've been a good boy I thought - haven't I ?

16 June 2012

09:00 hours abiraterone tablets taken as prescribed. 10:00 hours additional tablets taken as instructed. Internally, I am feeling coldish along with the hot flushes. This made for an uncomfortable morning. I continued shredding personal documents and packing my personal belongings in readiness. My partner Grace came over and we dined out and had a further chat about the move and intended expenditures.

In my mind things are not 100% between us and I decided to tackle this problem head-on.

Though our relationship is good I always felt that there were personal things unknown to me and I had no intention of moving in with a woman, I did not really know well enough. Tackling it head on proved to be difficult but I persisted and eventually I got a response from her. To be honest I was surprised but I learnt more about her in those few hours than I did in all the time I had known her, up to that point none of which were detrimental to our relationship. The real Grace came out and I knew then that I was being told the truth and furthermore, this woman knew then that our relationship was at stake and sought to preserve it.

Now I knew I could move in without the spectre of the past between us anymore. It was not my intention to make her cry or be mentally cruel, but I had a strong feeling that there were other factors not discussed and I had to know the truth. They do say the truth will set you free and it surely did set Grace this evening.

Even Josh had noted the change in my mood this evening and commented to his mum who then conveyed his sentiments to me. Kids are very perceptive when they get to know an adult. All I can try and do is to be there for him always.

17 June 2012

09:00 hours abiraterone tablets taken as described. 10:00 hours additional tablets taken as instructed. Grace visited my home today so I cooked Sunday lunch, which I was so glad to do as it is usually her that cooks so it made a refreshing change. Weather was nice, but the sweats were pouring off me as per usual. Finished packing more of my bags and after dinner we departed back to Grace's home where I spent a few more days Still unsure as to what I should do as regards moving, the independence in me is surfacing. It's kind of indicating that Grace and I both need to re-think. Early night as I feel quite tired.

18 June 2012

08:00 hours abiraterone tablets taken as prescribed. 09:00 hours additional tablets taken as instructed. Grace was unwell today so she took the day off I attempted to work on her ailments using some old Jamaican cold flu remedies passed down to me through my father. Dark rum, lemon, honey and garlic mashed up, combine this with an inhalation using bengay balsam this alleviated her blocked nasal passage and a certain amount of wellness immediately started to come back within her. Decided to be a bit of a handy man about the place and got busy with Garage door outside. Grace slept and rested for most of the day and by evening time she was almost like new and back to her old self.

19 June 2012

09:00 hours abiraterone tablets taken as prescribed. 10:00 hours additional tablets taken as instructed. Grace returned to work today feeling 90% better. I felt good in myself that I had made this old remedy "Never knock them. " I hated seeing her sick.

Received a call from my GP surgery requesting that I come and see him urgently. I was amazed that they had called however, concerned as I had just seen my GP last week. So the question running in my mind all day was "What Now?" what was so important that they would seek to request that I come and see my GP so urgently?

At first, I dismissed it as not urgent and made the appointment to see him for Friday 22nd, however on reflection and much thought, I changed my mind decided to make the appointment earlier for Wed 20th at 10:00 hours. My mind was ablaze with the question "what could it be now?" obviously I did not sleep well at all.

Contacted Grace and the kids and informed them all. Questions were asked by everyone to which, I could not answer. This upset me as I was now making all involved worried and scared and that was not my intention. Sometimes I believe it's best not to say anything until after the event. Early night to bed, still sweating though.

20 June 2012

07:00 hours abiraterone tablets taken as instructed. 08:00 hours additional tablets taken as instructed. Well, today was an extremely busy day at work and Grace attended my GP appointment with me for the first time. Today I was not alone and I can tell you that feeling was something very special indeed.

Previously, all my appointments have been virtually by myself and as I have stated before, I have been walking a very lonely and rocky path. Grace's presence made me feel that I was not alone and that I was somebody. Somebody also that was being cared for and loved. When I walked out today God placed an angel beside me to protect and care for me as well as report back to him. My first appointment today was with my doctor at 10:00 hours and we arrived there exactly on time and waited in the waiting room to be seen, after 15 minutes we were summoned into his office.

To our utter amazement all my GP wanted to do was to check up on me from the last appointment, which was less than seven days ago and the questions asked were such that this could have been done via telephone. We had driven from Harrow a journey taking just over an hour for an appointment, which lasted less than eight minutes. Grace had already warned me prior to going in not to lose my temper nor tell the doctor a few choice words as this could have an adverse effect on my medical file especially as I was about to change doctor surgery. Again, God had sent his angel to me for a reason unknown to me earlier but certainly later.

I was unhappy after leaving the surgery that my time had been wasted however; I had a more pressing appointment to attend. We headed towards the hospital for consultation with the doctor at 15.00 hours. Met with the doctor and discussed our list of questions that we had prepared. I allowed Grace to take the lead and I just sat back and listened and occasionally intervened, but for the most Grace did all the talking and note taking to the answers given by the doctor.

Clearly, a lot of the answers given by the doctor helped to alleviate much that was on our minds. It must be said that Grace conducted herself with intelligence and tact. We received all the answers to our questions and more and that was the most important thing as far as we were concerned.

Received a re-supply of my drugs along with an additional set of tablets, namely Potassium Chloride were given to me as one of the results showed that my potassium levels were slightly low. I felt very fatigued and sweaty as this had been a long day but for once I had someone on my side asking relevant and pertinent questions. This for us resulted in being able to further understand some of the side effects I was experiencing as well as what was going on with me medically.

The doctor confirmed that I am to stay on the stampede drug trials and that my next visit would be in six weeks' time. Medically all seems to be going in the right direction, I could see in Grace's face that she was a little happier and this made my day. I am without a doubt feeling good and just want the sweating to stop and go away. Once again I am indebted to Grace for her assistance in driving me to all my appointments, today had been extremely exhausting for the both of us.

21 June 2012

09:00 hours abiraterone tablets taken as prescribed. 10:00 hours additional tablets taken as instructed. Today I had to go back to the hospital to pick up my prescription that was not ready yesterday; my two daughters Celena and Lajade came along with me after which we had lunch. I have to say in my heart of hearts this was one of the most enjoyable times that I have had with these two daughters. Maybe it was the gaiety between the two of them, plus the love that exists between them. Though there is 11 years difference, that does not stop what clearly shows, are two close and loving sisters.

While in my presence, I could not do much more than stare and admire what I had bought into this world. I felt so proud also that I was able to go somewhere with these two divas.

Again sweating presented itself during the day along with a bout of fatigue. After picking up a prescription, I decided to stop at the trial nurse's office to introduce my two daughters to her, nice to be proud of your children and be able to introduce them publicly. Returned home around 19:00 hours and went almost immediately to my bed, as the week had taken its toll on my body. Called a journalist friend of mine and discussed the possibility of co-writing a book based around my professional career and cancer journey.

I have known him for many years and I had a desire quite some time ago to write a book even before my illness was diagnosed and felt maybe now was the right time. He suggested that we meet up to discuss the matter at length. It's funny, it's not until you get sick that you start to wonder how you will be remembered – maybe my book will help in that direction and reflect a true account.

22 June 2012

09:00 hours abiraterone tablets taken as described. 10:00 hours additional tablets taken as instructed. Decided that today was to be a day off my normal chores and business dealings.

I felt very tired and my body ached all over. My back seems to be playing up again and I need to be careful. I find that my reactions are still very much tip top and as such; I move very quickly and sharply at times forgetting all about my condition. Still sweating a lot, but slept until midday ignoring phone calls from whomever. Decided to give

Grace a treat by carrying out some home cooking and also setting a hot bath as she deserves it, so said so done. It was wonderful to see how much she appreciated it.

She needs to take it far more easily as she has a tendency to overdo things, especially after a hard day at work and then coming home to her family one of whom is sick but not an invalid. The sweats are proving a problem without a doubt more so when I am in the kitchen at any time the sweat just pours off me, something I had not experienced until now. I am concerned, especially as the summer months are just around the corner and I have a number of overseas work assignments that I have to attend where the climates are very warm indeed. Just wondering if I will overheat causing me other serious problems.

23 June 2012

09:00 hours abiraterone tablets taken as prescribed 10:00 hours additional tablets taken as instructed. Back pains are becoming more and more frequent along with the sweats. Today I carried out a few chores and helped Grace sort out a few external building issues.

Once again, I overdid my day out on the road and upon returning home around 18:00 hours I immediately went to my bed. Woke up around 12:20 hours took my medication, sent a few e-mails and finished writing a business security-training proposal for a government client. Eventually I went to bed at 02.30 hours and went out like a light and slept solidly.

24 June 2012

09:00 hours abiraterone tablets taken as prescribed. 10:00 hours additional tablets taken as instructed. Still feeling a bit tired so decided to have a lazy morning. Back pains are still plaguing me without any real ease up. Stayed at home to watch the Euro 2012 football game between England and Italy, what a waste of time to be honest, they got beaten on penalties. One issue that I am failing to make a note of is the frequency of my visits to the toilet to urinate, which is far more often than normal use. This occurs far more during the day than at night. Grace dropped me at home and stayed over. The fatigue along with the sweating played their parts in me going to bed early tonight.

25 June 2012

Contacted Doctors Surgery to change my hormone injection appointment to Wed 27th, at 11:00 hours, this was granted. Contacted my local hospital by e-mail as regards the letter received for an appointment with their Trauma & Orthopaedic unit. Email came back informing me that they were not aware of this appointment and that they would look into the matter. What's going on I ask myself, I mean no one discussed with me about this appointment even though, I was there 5 days previously.

I'm due to go to the hospital on Tuesday the 26th to pick up some more steroid tablets as enough was not administered to me when I picked them up last week.

I will drop a letter in for them to see and comment on further, I sweated buckets it's just like a tap turning on and off on my head, face and neck areas. It just won't ease up at all it seems. Rested and relaxed for most of the day and caught up with my symptom diary, e-mails and a few phone calls. At around 19.00 hours I found myself in bed, very early indeed to be honest, but I felt very tired indeed and could not stay up any longer.

26 June 2012

Realised this morning that last night I had not taken my late medication. 09:20 hours attended the surgery for my hormone injection, which was administered by one of the nurses interestingly a conversation struck up between us with regards to a product named

Arginine. Obviously, this was done unofficially but I was receptive to what was being offered. She was an African nurse with a very nice personality and caring nature and had noted before her on a computer screen all of my ailments.

Maybe many others would have objected, but the way she conducted herself intrigued me as I listened further with interest. At first she looked me up and down and I felt my sixth sense trip in it and a feeling of; I was being weighed up to see if I was approachable to converse with on a matter outside of usual medical boundaries. She noted I was sweating excessively and asked if I needed the fan, which I was appreciative of. She returned to the computer and looked at my details and then said straight out "I would like to give you a paper to read." I at first frowned until she said, "It's a medical product that I think will interest you and help you." Thereafter, I was all ears, the product was something she herself was taking however, she had also sent it over to her father who resided in Africa and who had diabetes as well as prostate issues.

She stated he telephoned her one-day and asked her what is this product that she had sent him as it is doing wonders that said alone perked my interest further. She related her sister's experience of being told that the lump in her sister's breast was cancerous and that the breast would have to be removed. To this day her sister's breast has not been removed due to the continual taking of the product Arginine which is a nitric oxide producer and high-potency anti-oxidant.

For another twenty minutes we conversed about alternative medicines, before the interruption of a phone call from the practice manager that a patient build-up was being created, whereupon we realised my injection still had to be administered. To be honest, I could only think that God had sent another of his angels to visit and advise me this morning regardless that I had not used the product as yet I knew an additional direction and path was being shown to me.

I thanked her and departed from the surgery with the new and invaluable knowledge running through my mind.

I felt our conversation expressed our disconnection with some aspects of modern medicine and the poisonous chemical introductions into our bodies that they can bring. My father taught me to try and understand that the old Caribbean medical remedies work far better than many modern medicines and I was always an advocate of using these remedies for myself and my children during our lifetime. Attended my next hospital appointment at 11:00 hours and picked up prescription for steroid tablets from the hospital pharmacy.

Met with trials nurse in the oncology department to verify the contents of the letter received stating Mr Samuels to attend hospital for an appointment with trauma and orthopaedics team on August 1st 2012 - I showed her the letter which seemed to mystify her but she decided to investigate further only to find out that the letter's information content was incorrect. Wrong hospital wing and wrong clinic unit. Anyway, I was then supplied with the correct information and departed the clinic unit only to get half way down the corridor when the nurse came running after me. I then found out wrong information was given. It turns out that the final correct information was that I was not after all seeing the trauma and the Orthopaedic team but my usual oncology consultant.

What concerned me most was the misinformation supplied. I could not help thinking that these were the people who have my medical care in their hands and they could not get a letter correct, beggars belief sometimes. Felt very tired and uneasy in my mind for some reason came home and rested for the rest of the evening.

27 June 2012

Woke up early feeling sickish could only put this down to the medication that I am taking. I also felt a few new pains through my body, but apparently from previous explanation, these were to be expected. The sweating was still very apparent as well as the return of the hot flushes, but then that was an expected side effect, due to the Prostap hormone received yesterday. Decided that I would relax today as drugs were starting to have varying effects on my mind and body, though this was compounded by the amount of travelling and stress I was undergoing.

Felt pains in my left arm and upper chest, sweating seems to have minimised however, I will keep an eye on it. Grace is keeping an eye on me though, which I don't have a problem with at all. It's funny, I have realised that I am receiving less and less contact from my so called friends at least those aware of my condition but my best friend Grace remains constantly by my side. I am still adamant that I will beat cancer my mind-set is firmly placed towards winning this, the hardest battle I have met to date.

I realised today that I want to spend at least the next 20 years with Grace; I want to spend and see my children grow up and have their own families. This particular feeling resonated with my late mother's wish, to at least live to see her children grow up. Life has a funny way of hitting you smack in the face at the least unexpected moments. I talked with the Lord today, like you would be talking on the phone to a friend and I asked him to watch over one of my daughters medical test results which are due tomorrow, for a lump found near her breast during a routine examination. Dare I say it God, please not my child also, oh please not my child, I could not bear that pain or anguish that would finish me off without a doubt. For most of the evening, I was not great company as my mind was on my daughter and her appointment.

28 June 2012

Woke very early felt slight pains in my left elbow and hand as well as left leg upper thigh, right leg above knee, right hand side (this one is usual and becomes more apparent after having the prostap injection), lastly chest area upper body. This morning I looked into Grace's face whilst she slept and noticed the blackness around her eyes were far more prominent than usual. Her skin tone is light and as such the blackness around her eyes was far more prominent than usual.

I know some of this is down to her work, but I can see it is also my illness that is stressing her out and this comes out in her face. It is times like these that I feel for her as well as I wish we were not so romantically involved. It would make walking away so easy but that is not to be. If it were I would do so in a flash, for her sake to minimise her stress level and mental strain that is evident.

Spoke to her about the above when she woke this morning and we agreed that a holiday was needed. She is due six weeks holiday in total because she has not taken any holiday leave this year so far, only a day here and there. What a gladiator she is at times, I don't know how she does it but she does.

Felt fairly okay though my lower back was still somewhat painful. 09:50 hours started feeling sickly in my stomach as well as my head feels light, I'm not in a good place at the moment. Stopped drinking milk and have replaced this with soya. Today I reflected again on the amount of pain the human body and mind withstand. Hardly a day passes where I do not undergo any sort of pain it is not the life I imagined, in my older years.

The weather was quite nice, but I was not sure if I should venture out as I needed to remain as cool as possible.

At around 11:00 hours I decided that I could not stay cooped up all day and ventured outside. The temperature was really hot for so early in the day. I have noticed that the texture of my hair has changed from the fine black hair that it was, to a coarse feeling type. I have shaved my head many times and it grows back coarser each time thereafter, I can only put this down to the medication, sadly another personal loss.

Trying not to let it worry me too much, as they say "the only easy day was yesterday." Those sentiments echo very well with me.

My daughter called me after her appointment at the Hospital reference lumps found near her breast. Good news, they are not cancerous and a great sense of relief was felt by me as she had been on my mind all day. It was noted that they found other further lumps, but all are very small and not cancerous. No further action is to be taken until they become larger. The weather became extremely hot and humid and I regretted my decision to venture outside, fortunately it was only locally, but the way I felt made me realise that I have to pay attention to and heed medical advice as regards staying out of the heat as much as I can.

I sweated so much that my handkerchiefs were totally soaked through. I also physically felt dried out with hardly any energy left in my body at all. It did not help matters that I had not drunk much water throughout the day. As the evening drew in my stomach still felt unsettled. Decided I would cook some steak as this would be quick and easy, but my mind is toying with the cessation of red meat next in my food cull. 23.00 hours ready for my bed as the weather had taken its toll on me today.

29 June 2012

Still felt rough on my stomach and a light-headed feeling in my head, which restricted my physical movements for the day. Grace dropped me home to make final arrangements for my move. It's funny how she noticed my mood and temperament whilst here at her home, clearly I am not happy in my home, goes without saying what to do.

A friend today commented on how well I look. I have to say external looks can be quite misleading people. If only they knew how I really feel. My days do differ in how I feel internally and how I managed physically, throughout the day. This also affects my mood to the point of self-awareness and I notice at times I have bounds of energy, walk, and move quickly, but in the same breath I linger and fall back to a tortoise pace. I just can't get to grips with that aspect, as I am use to being very energetic and agile. The sweats are still very apparent, but I must say they have become less frequent.

30 June 2012

My stomach feels a little wobbly along with my head. The sweats are still apparent, but not totally overbearing this morning. In general, this morning I felt that I was in a good place mentally. Staying firm with dietary change Soya milk now replacing skimmed milk. Decided to attend my grand niece's athletic meeting - at age ten, she is an aspiring sprinter in the making. The day itself was nice and along with my eldest daughter we arrived to watch her compete, unfortunately we arrived too late to see her compete and win her 100 metre sprint event in a time of 14.9 seconds and for her age that's quite good. She was again running at 16:00 hours in the sprint relays so we hung around for that event. Other family members were there also so it was a very nice family day along with the weather.

I felt so alone today and also watching my grandniece compete caused me to have a moment of nostalgia, as I once used to compete as an athlete some 34 years ago and I hasten to add was quite good, in fact very good. The relay event came and wow what a runner she is though she needs to understand baton-changing technique, but at aged ten, enjoying it is what it's all about.

I was quite proud of her additionally academically; she is learning to speak Chinese and doing well as she seems to be a very talented youngster. After the athletics meet we decided to all go out for a meal at TGI Friday's and that rounded off a nice day. Found that I was flagging towards the end of the evening and ended up in bed at 20:00 hours. I felt a little emotional earlier in the day, and a few tears were shed. Maybe the memories of what I used to do from a sporting perspective got the better of me, or maybe it was the side effect of the prostap injection.

1 July 2012

Felt a sharp pain in my left arm and left hand is slightly swollen. Do not feel at all good, a sickly feeling was felt in my stomach along with general bodily weakness is what I experienced. Rested virtually the entire day due to the sickly and weak feelings. During the evening, I sweated continuously for between three to four hours, consistently wiping my head and chest. Went out for a twenty-thirty minutes walk, to try and cool down, but the day was somewhat muggy day, so my attempt to cool down did not work. Forgot to mention that I urinated far more frequently than usual today.

2 July 2012

Felt groggy but not as bad as yesterday morning. Had a busy business day with a major meeting in London, with an overseas government representative. Still felt groggy throughout though. Received a telephone call reference the Arginine product and was given the all clear by my oncologist. My back was still playing me up and I need to make a firm decision as to what to do medically. This feeling of loneliness never seems to leave my side. Occasionally a friend may call, but I still feel so alone in my fight. I want to call and speak to people and let it all out, but my personal privacy stops me from doing so, so I stay alone and lonely. Can't wait for the day I move out and in with my partner Grace I'm sure it will change this mood that I feel.

I have arranged a special surprise night out for us both this weekend, I am quite sure that this will put a different slant on our relationship, this I am sure of.

3 July 2012

Well, another day and I just propped myself up in front of my computer wishing at times it could talk back to me and help me through my lonely days. Felt fairly okay today, stomach was not so groggy, but I still had that sickly feeling. Slept very well last night, though sweating still persisted, but not as bad as last week. Grace is coming over this evening to help finalise my move. I cooked us a nice meal. A friend of mine called me late and informed me that his ex-partner the mother of his children, died two weeks ago from cancer, even though she had gone into remission but the cancer came back and went to her liver.

My thoughts were clearly with my friend, however, he is unaware that I am currently a cancer sufferer and I felt that now was not a good time to tell him. I lay in bed and thought much about my friend and his ex-partner's situation, wandering if I could go the same route

4 July 2012

Woke in the early hours and felt a bit low in myself. My pillow was drenched with my sweats again, felt rather uncomfortable; this almost regular event is becoming unbearable. Grace and I had a heart to heart talk as regards her question to me "How do I feel about everything to date as relates my Cancer" I responded by saying having now had time to adjust to the news as well as to the impact on my life, I was now more adapt and felt that I was managing far better. Though I still struggle to understand my GP's statement that he believes I should be thinking short-term rather than long-term reference life expectancy.

Well, five months from that conversation, I was responding to my treatment. As Grace agreed short-term in her mind would be three to six months. She added a relevant point in that a discussion held with my oncologist that he did not class me as terminally ill thus my GPs comments are nothing to worry about at this stage, but one can't help thinking about it, you just can't ignore it, if you're a realist, as I am.

Grace reiterated to me my promise that I had made to her that I would be around for another ten years at least. I just smiled when she made the comment. Grace then told me how she admired my courage and determination and will to live, especially after seeing me in hospital back in April and witnessing the pain that I had been in and my determination then to live, she knew then that I was someone special who would survive. I must say that most of this would not have been possible if she were not part of my rehabilitation process. Our sexual intimacy was also a point of discussion to which I stated that yes the very core of my masculine identity had been taken away and that my dampened sexual libido worried me, in that could our relationship withstand a relationship where side-effects were 'lack of sexual interest'.

Grace urged me to remember that our relationship was based on the building of friendship first. Felt not so bad today though after a bit of physical activity in lifting boxes and moving items I was left puffing and slightly wheezing. Clearly I need to discuss all these matters with my doctors. I noticed a spasm that is occurring in my right hand where my middle finger closes up against my index finger, causing painful spasms; I need to keep an eye on this, as it is something new.

Tonight I sat back and listened to some music, namely the late country & western artist Jim Reeves. As a child growing up, I was introduced to his music and I have not strayed far from it into my adult years, in listening and collecting. Mum, Dad, thanks for allowing me to appreciate this kind of music, as it kept me during lonely moments and times of distress.

It also brought back memories of you both. You'll probably know that I'm very sick as I feel your presence at times watching over me and mine, during this period of my life. Thank you, thank you so much. It was a tearful evening I had but an enjoyable one if you follow my direction, but you need to be deep to do so, very deep indeed. Grace is a new chapter emerging in my life and I am of the opinion that this is the final stage for me in my search for a faithful and solid partner, I have what I want and what is good for me. Though the question remains of how long in terms of months and years that may be for remains to be seen.

I am the happiest I've been in a long while as tears fall down my face I truly realise the true meaning of Loving, Caring, Respecting and being cared for. It's funny that Grace and I have similar feelings, back in April when I was admitted to into hospital I thought I was going to die and she also thought my time had come. It takes my thoughts back to that day with a deepness like I have never had, where I was calling for my eldest daughter Celena as I lay on a trolley in A&E with those dear to me shedding tears around me. I could only think of her not being there as I felt my moment had come to die. I was conscious that she was on her way, travelling to the hospital to see me and I felt I had to hang on regardless of the pain to see her one last time. She would never have forgiven me if I had died before she arrived, Precious Memories.

5 August 2012

Woke early sweating as usual, just don't feel myself lacking that zest. Had an appointment in central London at 13:00 hours. Arrived back home at 17:00 hours, felt fairly okay and not overly sweating. Watched the T.V and then bam it all started to go wrong, once again a feeling of un-wellness came upon me like nothing I had experienced before; I can't really explain it other than to say I was not myself. What came over me could only be best described as a feeling of my inner body organs feeling cold and unwell.

I went and lay down to try and shrug it off. While lying on the bed, fully clothed I felt the sensation of hot one minute and then cold the next. I wrapped myself up in the duvet cover, but then I really started to feel cold, especially in the forearm area of both hands along with my chest. Being totally honest for the first time ever, I was scared of dying, I really was. I immediately texted Grace as to her whereabouts and also Celena and Lajade also to call me fearing the worst. Grace replied with a text saying '3' which I took to mean three minutes from home.

I texted her back saying baby hurry home ASAP. Lajade called and it was at that moment the feeling of un-wellness really accelerated and I began to shiver and shake uncontrollably. Lajade was still on the phone with me, was distraught and told me to call an ambulance at which the front door bell rang. With phone in hand and still conversing I attempted to get out of the bed, I swung both my legs over the edge of the bed to meet the floor and pushed upwards to become vertical and took one step towards the bedroom door which I never made. An excruciating pain emanating from the mid back area of my body, took over my entire body and I collapsed onto the floor in a heap and cried out in pain. As I lay crumpled I heard my daughter scream, as the phone fell to the floor from my hand.

While I lay there in a heap behind the door, I heard the bedroom door handle turn, as someone attempted to gain entry, but they could not, as I was blocking access. A voice shouted out to me. It was Grace. Once again, I found myself having to find the strength from somewhere, to push myself up and away from the door to allow her access. I still to this day do not know how I managed to do it I really don't. Once she had gained entry she bent down and assisted me to the bed edge where I propped myself up against the bed headboard.

At this point I realised that the phone line to my daughter was still open and asked Grace to pass me the phone. I engaged in a few seconds of conversation with her to reassure her I was ok and that Grace was here and would assist me now. I told her to call Celena and explain what had occurred and for her to call me. Grace immediately took my pulse (78 slightly irregular but strong) and temperature (36.4) and inspected my hands for any telltale medical signs. She then got me to sit up properly and re-encounter what had taken place the previous fifteen minutes, which I was able to do so. She then made me urinate into a bowl and checked my urine, which indicated that my glucose level was abnormal (+++) all else was negative. It was at this stage she wanted to call an ambulance.

I refused her request, I know, hard-headed and stubborn, but the thought of going back to a hospital that I did not care for aghast me. I can only tell you that I hate attention of any sort. Eventually, she contacted the on-call oncologist at my hospital, which was around 20:00 hours and relayed what had occurred. Having heard the facts the doctor requested that I make my way immediately to A&E where he would arrange for me to be seen as my symptoms suggested an infection of some sort.

Before I left for the hospital my pulse was taken again at 19:50 hours (90 strong but irregular). Grace had just come home from a full day at work and now had to head towards an A&E department. This was a one hour drive away from where we resided. To say I felt unhappy was an understatement, but she did it and grateful is far from the appropriate word to use. Once again, my angel was by my side.

Upon my arrival at A&E department, it was as if a major incident had happened, almost every seat was taken and a minimum of four hours wait loomed. We reported to the assessment sister and I produced my cytotoxic chemotherapy card, which seemed to act like an American Express black card. To those of you who are in the know I need not explain, to those not it's the card that makes the AmEx platinum card look like a Tesco's points card. I did not even have time to sit down and get comfy before my name was called. Less than 5 minutes I believe.

I was taken into accident and emergency, into a room not a cubicle at which both Grace and I looked at each other with an expression of WOW the NHS aren't so bad after all. Within ten minutes, a male nurse attended to me and did the vampire bit again, my bloods were taken. Ouch, it hurt this time and I mean really hurt as a needle was inserted into my left arm. So within fifteen minutes of entering the hospital here I was well underway to being medically assessed and loving it.

The oncologist S.R medical doctor attended and I explained myself again to him, as he was the doctor I spoke to before leaving home to attend A&E. Further tests were carried out blood sugar 8.8; BP 157/91; temperature 36.9, Nil blood, no raised white cells, and urine nil.

No infection was apparent, as there were no clinical symptoms. So all in all everything seemed to be okay. Having had all these tests it seemed apparent that things were a bit of a mystery. Then in his presence, wham, my lower back gave way and I started to collapse. I had to be aided by the doctor, and Grace to the couch, which alarmed the doctor and a medical note was made in my file with an urgency placed on this to be addressed sooner rather than later as my next hospital appointment was not until August 1st. The doctor indicated that he would arrange for this to be bought forward and then referred me for an x-ray, before I departed the hospital. The drive back home took us an hour and I recalled saying to myself "God this day I was so appreciative of you sending your angel to watch over me and furthermore, that nothing too sinister seemed medically wrong with me."

Ladies and gentlemen, I have to say I was a player in my younger days and still a bit of a player as I got older, but I can honestly say that Grace has shown me such love, care, and attention that even the thought of cheating on her or allowing her to feel second rate never ever crosses my mind. As I stated before, I have found my life long soul partner at long last.

6 August 2012

Felt very tired today due to the late finish at the hospital this morning 02:00 hours to be precise, decided to take it easy today.

Contacted the Hospital oncology department to update them about the accident and emergency visit. My August 1st appointment has now been moved forward to July 11th due to concerns about the back pain and management thereof. Just feeling groggy and sickly in my stomach and of course, the sweats are still having a field day with my body.

Also had some weak feelings going on in my legs. Grace and I have a date on Saturday and if I have to crawl into it, I will. This was arranged a few months back and it's going to be special so it's going to be a case of mind over matter. Grace looks concerned about what's going on with me, but she does not know how much my inner strength will prevail.

7 August 2012

Left home early to get to the barber's in preparation for tonight's surprise night out with Grace. Whilst I went to the barber's, she was at the hairdresser's. I came home and prepared my going out clothes before she got back. We had asked a photographer friend of Grace's – Marcia - to come along and take some pictures of the two of us, which she duly did.

These were great inside and outside of the home and they added to the whole evening as well as to a certain indirect intimacy that was missing in the home; 'Our photo'. The car arrived at 18:30 hours and off we went on our surprise night out. Well, at least for Grace not me as I had arranged it all. We arrived at 19:35 hours at Victoria embankment to board a boat called the symphony a glass topped boat, which carried out river dinner cruises. I had arranged this surprise back in May.

Elite dining tickets, five course menu with music. This classy event was fully booked but I had pre-arranged window seats for the night. We both looked and dressed impeccably for the evening and in my mind were apart from the rest of the other diners aboard without a doubt. Grace looked everything that a Queen should look and act like tonight and as we walked hand-in-hand to our table, we could feel the roving and admiring eyes upon the pair of us. Having been seated at a table the night began.

A photographer came along and introduced himself to us whose services were included in the price of the tickets I had purchased; this allowed us to have a few photographs taken on board the boat.

Grace's face was nothing short of a lady totally in love with the attention of the event and the night. I have never seen my partner's eyes, glitter so like tonight. Love was truly at our table tonight and the whole preparation aspect of the event was truly worth it to me and most definitely to her.

Even the photographer indicated he was looking forward to taking our pictures, as we looked like a special couple. Little did he know that one of us was very special indeed. Two other separate diners came across to our table and asked if we would like our picture taken together with our own digital camera that we had bought with us and were intermittently clicking at each other. Some even commented on how well we looked together along with gaiety and laughter emanating from our table. Tonight was in celebration of being together (July 20 for one year). It was also my way of saying a special and massive thank you to Grace for all that she had done for me to date and more. She cried as I spoke those words to her, but she also knew that not only was I lucky to be here, but also that I may not be here again in the months ahead. The night was so memorable that even I became emotional since I walked in with a Queen and walked out with an Empress. I'll never forget the look in her eyes and the photographs taken, as they say the cameras never lies as our photographs showed two people truly in love. Our lives had changed forever and Mr&Mrs. Samuels were born.

I asked Grace to be dressed like a Queen for the night she excelled herself and came as empress divine. With all pictures taken, fed, watered, inebriated, and bloody tired we returned home and hit our beds at 12:30 kissed each other a few times and were out for the count. She was mine and I hers and the issue of me with cancer were far from both our minds. Our love had been captured for all to see and our relationship cemented beyond a doubt for all to see. During the night, I felt not so good, but considering the evening we had, it was not surprising so I slept on until the morning.

8 August 2012

My daughter Lajade came over today for dinner, which was just so lovely, she and Grace get on so well and that makes it so much more wonderful. She is elated that her dad is moving closer to where she resides, this means so much to her. My life was spent around travelling and some of my children did not grow with me, nor understood what or why I did what I did from a professional career perspective.

Now aged 20, Lajade seems to be far more understanding in that area. We are close, in fact very close and this makes for a wonderful father/daughter relationship. She stands at 5ft 9 and walks strong and proud and is so beautifully combined with a terrific smile and personality. You just warm to her when you see and meet her. That's why I keep our relationship so special, and anything that I can do to enhance it further, I would do. We spoke in-depth as to how I was feeling and what the future medical consultation appointments would look to deal with.

I also found out that her grandfather is in hospital suffering from cancer. This saddened me as the two closest people from a male perspective in her life were suffering from cancer, what a bummer for her to deal with at her age. My eyes welled at this news and my only words to her were "Both dad and granddad have cancer how sad" to which she nodded. Again a reason for me to live and survive this.

19 August 2012

Strange feeling waking up in a foreign country, but I felt well today so far, but apprehensive as I know should anything go wrong medically that I am overseas. I had to carry out a security risk assessment visit here today in Nice, France and then return back home to the UK tomorrow. The car picked us up at 11:30 hours for site visit.

Upon arrival at the site location it became clear that what lay ahead was no easy task. It turned out that the site in question was half of a mile walk downhill from a cliff top path and then the same distance back uphill in 31º C. Well, I have to report that I completed this extremely physical and arduous task, but only just. Walking down to the site was not so bad, though I found I was over-striding and placing a strain on my back at times. To complicate matters further there was a lack of oxygen as the area was overshadowed by trees, shrubbery and plant life.

By the time we reached the bottom our bodies and shirts were totally soaked, and I was in a right state. Luckily, I wore a light shirt, which allowed air to reach my body. Having completed the mission the daunting walk back uphill faced me and my brother who was in attendance. Mentally, I prepared myself in the old military style of left, right, left, right, left, right, long strides then short strides and that worked for the first 200m. Then the heat and humidity struck and breathing became difficult as did walking. The muscles in my legs were fighting hard to work, but with the lack of oxygen and the muscle wastage/fatigue I had suffered over the past months they were close to collapse.

I hardly had any strength to continue pushing me onwards and upwards. Other people in the vicinity were finding it hard also but to my amazement, I did make it back to the top without further incident, to the waiting vehicle. Drenched not soaked was how I stood, propped against the car with the driver looking in awe. They say "the race is not always won by the swiftest – rather slow and steady steps will still get one to the finish and VICTORY". Clearly, this definitely was no race I was in. It was a physical test of my endurance, strength, stamina, and determination to overcome another barrier in front of me, and I succeeded. The thoughts that raced through my mind, were that of are you mad. I have cancer and went and exerted myself beyond the realms of physical possibilities and medical advice to remain cool and not to over exert myself.

My breathing was rapid and fast, but I couldn't help but admire myself at the achievement. Upon entering the vehicle the driver instinctively knew that what was needed, the air conditioning came on and man did I lap that up. But not for long as my wet clothing were sticking to my skin and I became fearful of catching a serious cold, so we had to head back to the hotel for me to dry off and take a change of clothing. My report was compiled and completed that evening without further incident and an early night was had.

20 August 2012

The flight back to the UK from Nice took us approximately 1 hour and 20 minutes, I felt a little claustrophobic on the journey back with a clogging feeling in my throat. What a feeling of total relief when we landed at Heathrow airport. I had carried out the tasks requested of me and had managed my first assignment in months. Grace met us at the airport and was elated to see me though, only 24hours had passed, she knew I had gone through an exhaustive time; little did she know the rest at the story.

A lovely Sunday roast dinner was laid on by her and much appreciated by me. Felt very tired and in pain after dinner and a very early night was where I headed to after dinner. Much of the pain was in my legs, especially my thighs, but other than that nowhere else, I suppose only to be expected.

21 August 2012

I was up early today, as I had to attend a funeral, that of my daughter's grandfather who unfortunately passed away from cancer. I did not feel my best today and that's maybe because I was jet-lagged somewhat. The service went well without any hitches though, I felt very emotional throughout, I could not help thinking this could so easily have been me.

My eyes at times were so watered that I could not see the service programme and hymn sheets to sing the songs, I just ended up humming. When a favourite hymn of mine was sung "God be with you till we meet again" which I knew the words to off by heart I found myself resolved of memory. To be honest, my body and mind had been subjected to much over the past 72 hours.

Found myself sweating profusely during the service, which made me feel rather uncomfortable, even though the windows were open in the church.

At times, my legs became lifeless especially with the standing up sitting down type of service that it was. Once the service was finished, I headed home for a well-deserved sleep. Don't really remember much more until late in the evening when Grace woke me up for dinner, after which I headed straight back to bed and slept like a baby. Well, glad that Tuesday is a rest day, even though a text came through offering me a security assignment commencing at 07:00 hours for a 36 hours shift for a sum of £350 it didn't appeal to me as much as my sleep, plus it was somewhat light in £ so it got a refusal.

22 August 2012

Woke up several times during the night to urinate. This is an ongoing occurrence for me. Still felt some discomfort in my groin, which seemed to bring on the desire to urinate. The day was fairly nice, slightly clammy, but none the less nice. Felt unwell today, felt very tired, lacking energy and generally yucky. Changed appointments for today to Thursday.

Grace is off work for 2 weeks holiday and we have tried to see if we could get away for a week, but either the costs are prohibitive or the flights returning just don't meet our required dates. I do feel that my condition plays a part in this also, in that we are limited to where we can go as I cannot take long-haul flights, so two hours is the maximum. I felt so unhappy that this precludes matters and today I discussed it at length with Grace. Told her maybe she should take a holiday by herself away from me. She has been my rock and pillar, but I just feel she needs time away from me for herself and to re-charge her batteries.

She's not having any of it so it was a pointless suggestion. It's a point that I'm sure we will come back to at some stage later. Decided in the end to go away to Gambia in the first week of November. In the interim, we are just going to throw some things into the car and drive to somewhere in the UK. No real idea of where, but we will sort that out once we are in the car. Sounds kind of exciting to be honest – just drive in some direction and find a place of interest and rest for a few days there.

Grace has actually been off work for a few days is working wonders already, she already looks less stressed and the blackness around her eyes minimised. She's looking really good these last few days, makes me so happy, but also tells me that a 2-3wks holiday in a tropical climate would also do her the world of good. Went out for a meal tonight, it's too hot to cook and I'm pissed off with food eating in general, so Chinese it was. A nice evening out we had, though I just found myself fighting to keep back the tears to the point of clenching my fists to hold them back.

These are the moments when I feel so at a loss and vulnerable; it's a feeling of no control in my life.

It's funny as I write these notes, Grace is nattering away at me and mentally I am in a different place. As I write these words she comments,

"You are not interested in what I'm saying are you?"

Actually, Grace I'm so in a different world you could not imagine when I write these words, I hear you but I don't hear you. Our evening was spent cuddling up in bed watching two movies and laughing. Something we have not done in a while. It was just so lovely to re-kindle a special moment.

23 August 2012

Still urinating in the early hours of the morning about five times between midnight and 06:00 hours. Felt a little woozy this morning not fully steady on my feet, this is something that comes and goes and I attribute to one of the side effects. Arginine supplement taken as instructed on the label. Had a busy day today with meetings in Central London along with some shopping items. Sweating is still occurring and my handkerchief was soaked after using it to mop my forehead and scalp. Managed to get all of what I set out to do today, though I felt woozy as I headed home. Mail received from the department of pension's reference my Disability Living Allowance application. The application was denied – What have you got to have wrong with you before you are entitled to benefits in this country?

Well, I have news for you guys I am not giving up so easily and will appeal the decision. I have not fought cancer like I have for the past eight months to give up, you don't know me yet, but you will – You sure will.

I deserve it and I am entitled to it. I'm not one of those that does not. The frequency of me urinating is becoming an issue, as I cannot travel too far from home without the need to use a toilet.

Further, I am not having regular bowel movements and when I do I find that I am straining. I must make sure that I point this out to the consultant on my next visit. Within myself today I felt highly emotional once again and the need to cry was still very much apparent. No real pain in my lower or upper back areas to complain about.

24 August 2012

Felt off-key today. My body balance and coordination were not in sync. My stomach felt as if it could do with a clear out. Urinating frequently as per usual, drank loads of liquid throughout the day though, but not much water. Emotionally, I felt weepish and slightly low in mood, not sure what the reason was but as usual, I just felt that way. Glad that we did not plan to go away for the bank holiday, as I would not have been physically or mentally up to it or good company.

Still pushing along and ahead with business projects, hoping that these will lead to fruition and big bucks. I have noticed that watching T.V programmes that are slanted to family dramas and parental unity that I get very emotional and fight back the tears when I watch them. I find that I am reflecting a great deal these days about my life and my children, when these programmes are shown. My right foot seems to be swelling a lot of late, especially in the ankle area, even though the weather has calmed down in terms of heat intensity.

In a bid to alleviate this issue I must try and keep my foot in an upright position far more often.

Finished outstanding work project synopsis this now leaves me freer to concentrate on relaxing. I feel that the stress of working so much is causing me moments of pain, especially in the lower and upper back areas. I get spasm shooting pains, which seem to be more apparent when I am working than not working.

25 August 2012

Grace and I had a lay in today and did not venture out of the bedroom until almost 13:00 hours. Carried out some light work around the house today, but sweated like a pig for it though. Found myself shuffling around the house for the later part of the day. I did not feel right in my mind.
The constant urinating is still causing me concern and I need to have a discussion with my GP as soon as I can. Grace and I watched TV this evening and at around 23:00 hours I took my late medication only to observe Grace burst out in tears as I was taking them. It really must be so hard for her to see me, day after day and night after night, having to take these life saving drugs regimentally.

I recalled saying baby at least I'm alive because of these tablets. She just lay next to me with her head in my lap and looked up at me and said nothing. I pray each day for her and her son Josh to continue to be able to deal with all what I have to go through, as well as should I die that the impact will not be so devastating to them. When I look at Grace, I still see an angel. Have you ever seen an angel? Well, I have, as I have said repeatedly. She is right before me, and her name is Grace Johnson and God sent her to care for me, I wonder if you have an angel looking over you, if so you will understand.

26 August 2012

Felt better than yesterday though not 100%, but better none-the-less. Daytime sweats seem to have subsided as opposed to nights. Went out for a nice walk today around the West Harrow recreational ground, which gave my legs a much-needed workout as I have not been out of the house for a few days. Still feeling that there is a muscle wastage issue going on with my legs, I am most definitely feeling weak in my legs and feel that at times they just feel like they can't support me and the feeling of collapse lingers.

Nonetheless Grace and I still had a nice slow walk through the park. My daughter Celena came over to see me it was so nice to see her, especially as she is the eldest, but also the fact that she drove a fair distance to see me. We spent a few hours together and had a real laugh about a few special photos of her taken many years ago. I decided that I would create a special album of my children's photographs, Celena and I wrestled about a few pictures, which she was not in favour of. However, what she did not realise was that these were the photos that gave me great pleasure and pride, these were the photos that when no one was around that I would look at and would give me hope to get through my day and illness.

As I don't see them every day these pictures were a substitute for the next best thing.

Emotionally, I felt very negative again; I still am not sure why I'm having these mood swings. The last few days my mind had to deal with a funeral, thoughts of dying, my own will arrangements, all these were things on my mind. Many times I have found it hard to concentrate and write a full page, other times it all just rolled off the pen nib onto the paper. I realised this week that there is really only a handful of people in my life giving me constant attention, friendship, love and most importantly care.

My mind falls on a few words of a poem that befits them:
"Many the friends who will walk by your side when you travel a smooth, even road, but few who remain when it's rocky and steep and you struggle to carry your load."

I found these few words to be the most appropriate and best suited for those in my life. Each day it has been about enlightenment, finding myself, reliving my past and in doing so I found the real me. The therapeutic value of writing cannot be measured, as the distance is never ending. It has only been seven months since my diagnosis and I am realising that I have much more to write. I trust in God to allow me the strength and time to write.

27 August 2012

Bank holiday today in the United Kingdom and the weather was not bad, though muggy and caused me to sweat a lot. I am noticing internal changes to my bodily system, which clearly have been a slow process. My lower and upper back regions are rarely painful though, at times slightly stiffer. Also noted that emotionally, I am much calmer and there is less tendency for me to resort to tears for no reason.
The frequency of urination is increasing and this does not ease up night or day (though during the daytime I tend to urinate more frequently). We spent the day lying around the home and online attempting to book a mini break in the UK somewhere, we are still undecided, especially as everywhere is booked up but we are persisting.

28 August 2012

Felt a little fatigued and generally unwell, I sweated a lot last night but not heavily. I still have to remind myself that this is only the seventh month, since I have been diagnosed and in that period of time I've gone through much. I am a far distance from a full recovery or at least remission. I assisted Grace at home today with moving clothing, bags and furniture around as we have a builder coming in tomorrow to carry out some work in the home. The place is going to be messy due to drilling for extra air vent holes which are needed in the home. I did not feel over exerted after physically moving things around; in fact it did me the world of good.

29 August 2012

I felt good today, though slightly unstable on my feet and stumbled when I walked at times during the day. I now believe that this is primarily due to the medication, which is causing me to experience this roller coaster feeling that I am undergoing. Our day was quite busy in and out of the home, eventually arriving back home around 20:00 hours. My body just felt totally void of energy and just fit to drop which I did, into my bed. We decided that we would take a mini-break this weekend in the City of Bath, in the west of England. I could see Grace was getting very downhearted that this might not happen, especially as she was due to go back to work the following week after a two-week break. We decided we would get all our work done by early on Thursday and then see if there were any last-minute.com deals around, a little break was better than none at all.
30 August 2012

We had an early start today managed to finish all our work and business affairs by 15:00 hours. I felt tired for most of the day, not knackered unlike how I would have felt a few weeks ago. Grace investigated a lastminute.com deal and got us a weekend deal in the City of Bath. The elation on her face was almost like her recent surprise diner cruise. It was evident that she needed the break, as the stress was starting to show on her face.

Grace needed it far more than me even if it was only for two and a half days. We decided that we would also visit the Roman spa mineral baths whilst we were there so as to take full advantage of the healthy option that would benefit both of us. We packed a small bag for a few days and, as we were going to drive, we retired early to bed.

31 August 2012

Felt good mentally, though a little apprehensive about our road journey today, but then that's just me. Personally, I would have preferred the train; it would have been far safer and less physically demanding on both of us. Though the advantage with the car would be that we could pack more than we needed or required and freely move around the city and its surroundings.

We departed from home and Grace drove the entire journey. Hats off to her, as I did not feel up to doing it. The journey took us about three and a half hours with a one-hour layover. Imagine if I had driven how I would have felt. I recalled doing these types of journeys in the past with ease, but not anymore. I felt that my confidence to drive had taken a hit. This to me was due to a twitchy nervousness that I had developed over the past months. At times when I drove, I would get twitches in my head and with this the nervousness came on. It got to the point of where I thought I might pass out or have a heart attack.

I never actually confided this to Grace, as I did not want to worry her additionally but I did go and see my doctor, who examined me but could not find anything immediately wrong. He warned me if it continued that I may have to inform DVLA which meant that my licence could be suspended. We arrived safe and sound and checked into our hotel which was not the busiest, but was nice and clean, quiet and just what we needed. Grace's face made me feel so happy as she was just completely chilled to the room and its surroundings. As the evening was drawing in fast, we decide to eat out in the town centre. That was a fifteen minute walk away, which allowed my legs to stretch and be rid them of the twinges I was having. After we came back to the hotel, and my medication was taken and two very tired people were out for the count in less than five minutes.

1 September 2012

We both had a very good sleep this morning, but what would you have expected from lying on a large four-poster bed. Grace looked well and rested also. This mini-break, though late, has worked out very well in our favour and I had to thank Grace for her persistence in finding something.

After breakfast, we ventured out into the wonderful city of Bath, and did the tourist thing, walking around the city, which I found to be very quaint, and to my taste and liking. I personally had not been there in over a decade and it had changed immensely. The afternoon was spent at the Roman mineral baths where we indulged in the rejuvenation of our minds, spirits and bodies. It was a blessing from heaven – indoor spa pool – hot tub with scent; outdoor spa pool and restaurant were all indulged in.

The whole experience has added to our lovely weekend so far and could be seen in both of our faces and felt in our bodies. For me also a moment of nostalgia was re-visited in my mind. I recalled as a young boy, my father doing a similar journey but by himself. He had a few weeks off work and we were at school at the time, so he decided that he would go away by himself for a few days, which he did, he took the train and spent a few days in Bath.

When he returned all he could talk about was this place in Bath called, the Roman mineral baths that he visited along with some pictures of the city of Bath. The look on his face was the look I saw on Grace's face.

So if the feelings I was feeling then were anything to go by, then he must have had a real good and rejuvenating time. The only thing was that he caught some hell from my mother for doing it though, as I recall the price for cleansing the inner soul I suppose. Tonight we ate Italian, which was very nice, cosy and romantic, but isn't that always the case with a nice Italian restaurant? In myself, I felt well and Grace looked a picture of her former self at times, especially no coughing or sneezing in the early morning, which I felt were telltale signs of the environment we lived in. There is much to say about living in the countryside. Once again, upon arriving back at the hotel we were out for the count once our heads hit the pillows and bed.

2 September 2012

Well, today being Sunday was our checking out day. Got to say that I did not look forward to doing so as our weekend had been so wonderful. Felt fairly well this morning. Though we did much I did not feel exhausted, nor fatigued just relaxed and at ease. I know Grace felt the same way also because she told me so. Ahead of us was a two and a half hour drive. I now felt that I could attempt this journey and volunteered to drive us back home. I felt a bit nervous as this was the longest drive that I was about to perform in many months.

There were a few times that I panicked whilst manoeuvring but I kept it together. My back did not even cause me any discomfort during the drive back at all, nor did I suffer from any other muscular complaints. We did not even stop for a break on our journey back, so you can understand how well I managed the journey. I was chuffed to bits.

Back in London, back to the smog, already missing the city of Bath. Though I personally would not reside there I most certainly would visit there again without a doubt. We ventured to bed earlier as Grace returns to work tomorrow, I feel for her as it's plainly on her face that she does not want to go back and could you blame her. As for me the reality of the situation was that for a few days, I managed to escape my usual surroundings, and I was again able to forget about my illness, and spend quality time with Grace but, in reality we were about to start all over again, life sucks at times doesn't it?

25 October 2012

It's been a while since I last wrote in my journal, in fact just over six weeks. I now feel compelled to start again as much has happened in the last six weeks that is worthy to mention. Today I attended my appointment at for my six weekly check-up. Grace and I arrived around 12:30 hours whereupon I attended the blood test unit and had my blood taken. The good thing was that I had a red sticker applied to my request form, which allowed me to jump the queue, which was a very handy thing I must say. Two vials of blood were taken from my left arm, which over the last six weeks has taken a battering leaving bruises and becoming very painful when further attempts are made to insert a needle to take more blood.

Today was an exception, though with the needle entering the left vein very easily and the blood flowing out into the vials. After the procedure, I had to wait two hours for my actual consultation to obtain the new PSA results and other blood related results, as well as my recent bone and CT scan results. So overall today was a very important day for results and I felt extremely apprehensive as did Grace. We had talked the night before on how we both felt about what these results meant to each other and interestingly enough, we concluded with saying-that having seen my PSA drop from 509 in January 2012 to 0.28 we wondered if we could see a similar situation internally that was on par with the PSA level drops.

I saw in my partner's eyes how much this meant to her as over the last six weeks her commitment, love, nurturing, caring attitude were all evident in my overall fight against this disease. More so I had gone through much pain and anguish these past weeks to the point of wanting to walk out on our relationship over a very stupid argument. The hurt I saw in her eyes that day when I said I was leaving will haunt me for a long time, as will the look on her face when she came home from work last night that countered the above intention.

Anyway, it didn't happen so we moved onwards and upwards. We arrived at the hospital on time and waited in the waiting room for my appointment. I noticed the conversation between us was minimal and an air of apprehension existed as we waited. Our wait felt like an eternity, as the clocked ticked away to our appointment. Many things passed through my mind as I sat waiting, especially as I looked around us and thought about other people in attendance and their suffering and the different stages that they were at. I wondered how much pain these people had undergone in their fight and struggle. If it was anything like mine, my heartfelt sympathy was with them and their families at that very moment in time. The one thing that I did notice was that almost everyone had someone in attendance with him or her. Whether as a parent, partner, wife or husband or community volunteer there was someone with them. Those that did not have someone with them I found to have a certain look about them, their facial features and expressions gave way to the lonely road they were travelling and I felt for them, for their go I if not for the Grace of God. Excuse the pun but its intended, Grace and God were working together to help me through this illness to a cure.

At 15:25 hours the doctor approached the waiting room door and called to Grace and I and we got up and greeted him at the waiting door and exchanged pleasantries. Personally speaking, I applaud this method of acknowledging patients it's professional, courteous and humane. The three of us walked down the corridor towards his office, but before we got there, he turned sideways to Grace and me and said I have some good news for you. I turned to Grace and gave her a knowingly look that my PSA level had dropped again and she smiled in a similar manner.

We entered his office, sat down, and he immediately revealed that my new PSA level was 0.19 indicating a further drop though, not as

150

significant as previous drops nonetheless a drop from the last reading of 0.28 to 0.19, which was very good indeed. This suggested to me that I was very close to the bottoming out figure and 0.19 is as dammit almost 0.00.

Grace smiled at me in such a way that the news of what was in her heart exploded onto her face on hearing the results, but nothing like what came to the reading of the next set of results. My scans had shown that the lymph lesions showing at the base of my lungs had all gone in fact the actual word used by the doctor was 'disappeared'. The lymph lesions at the base of my skull, in the area of my left side sixth rib and the L2, L3, and L6 areas of my back had significantly been reduced all due to the treatment of the abiraterone tablets.

The only negative issue was there remained a tumour type in my right groin of equal size as shown previously. Now to be honest, this news was such that the elation from my partner manifested itself in a heartfelt clench of my left thigh as well as a smiling face that lit up like London's, Oxford Street Christmas tree lights. The funny thing was though, was that I did not have the same elated feelings, nor did I really smile or jump for joy when the PSA or scan results were read out. Cool, calm, and collected was maybe a better description of my mood. I did not know what my reason was for my almost emotionless actions, other than maybe I knew that we had only travelled a short distance on this cancer journey and I feared much, much, more was to come before I could blow the trumpets of success.

Even my glucose level reading was 8.6 and considering that a month ago I was at a staggering 29 this was another major achievement and reduction in my health results. What was evident, though was that the steroids that I had been taking over the many months had affected my diabetes and resulted in frequent high blood sugar readings. Having attended my GP and been given metformin along with a strict diet had helped to bring my levels down to safety.

All other blood results given were all within normal ranges. A point to mention was that my scan showed that my right humorous was found to be rounded and as such no reason could be given to this reported state. On questioning the consultant, he answered that he had no idea as to what this meant which, actually was frustrating and we were left unclear to this part of the diagnosis. With all results in and questions raised, we made our official request for a transfer from my local hospital to Mount Vernon Hospital, which is based in Rickmansworth, Hertfordshire.

The transfer request was now made and we were informed that the process could take about two weeks after the senior oncologist at Mount Vernon hospital was contacted and had confirmed that there was room in their stampede drug trial programme for me. With that said the only thing left was for my blood pressure to be taken by the research nurse, which the reading taken was 145/83 with a pulse of 83. This concluded my visit to this clinic and actually my care with this hospital. The only additional thing to say was that it was confirmed that during the summer months I had been undergoing the abiraterone arm of the programme that I was the only patient to be signed to that arm of the trials programme in that hospital. I found this strange but who am I to argue as it has so far worked for me. I only wish that others could be afforded the same at an early stage of their diagnosis. I move on and hopefully to full recovery, nothing less will suffice.

My family, friends and most importantly Grace have played significant parts in my treatment and recovery over the past six weeks. Without them, I could not have done this, I have to admit to wanting to give up, and indeed more. My state of mind took me to a level that I never could have imagined. When you stand on top of a high building balcony just remember it's not as easy as you may think to take your life.

The streets that I walk alone day and night are my world, but I am without a doubt blessed and continue to be blessed. I was saddened today to learn of the death of church pastor Stephen Ramos. He had prayed for me when I attended his church in south London a number of months ago and he had visited me when I was hospitalised earlier in the year. I recall his words. God had told him when he initially had prayed for me, that I would be okay and even on a second occasion that he had prayed again for me God told him again, I have told you that you need not worry about him, this man Alfred will be well.

Pastor Ramos died of a brain haemorrhage in the early hours of today and I will never be able to see him again, RIP Pastor, RIP. It's so funny having attended his church in south London a few months before and finding myself in tears after being asked to introduce myself to his church congregation. I felt a deep loss at his death and sincerely extend to his family my deepest sympathy, because he surely was a man of God. Now I had to maintain a closer relationship with God so that I did not need to look for an interpretation of his word through someone else. If the truth be told my sisters Doreen and Valentina were still around.

My recovery is heading in the right direction, though again it is early days, as the trials are for a period of two years in total and we are 17 months away from the end of that term. The worst issue for me right now is the continuing sweating that I am experiencing, caused by the hormone injection prostap, which I receive every three months though this is a noted side-effect of the injection. Only since the last injection have I started to sweat every day profusely.

As the winter months draw in my concern is one of catching my death of a cold, especially as the weather temperature had dropped suddenly over the last twenty-four hours to a chilling 4° Celsius and my body really felt it. Though I must say it does not matter if it's hot or cold weather, I still sweat profusely.

A few times over the last few weeks, my mind has found itself back at the beginning of my cancer journey when I was first diagnosed. I have never been a gambler, but overcoming the odds was my aim then. I recall telling myself days later it may be stormy now but it cannot rain forever, every thunderstorm is followed by a rainbow. My sickness has motivated me to live and try and lead a normal life and make it to the next day. I needed to prove that having hope and inspiration could prove the notion that there was life after my illness and treatment. Grace came home tonight and while eating dinner looked over to me for an extended period without saying anything. I caught her gaze and questioned why she looked at me so in-depth, whereupon she said,

"I am just trying to understand how you get through each day. How do you keep doing it?"

I replied with the words, "I just do babes, I just do."

You see adversity introduces us to ourselves and in doing so, I have had a very long, deep and meaningful discussion with myself, not just simply on one occasion but many, as it's a recurring theme until changes were made within.

In addition, my family played a significant part in that process, especially with the advent of modern technology text messaging.

Chapter 5 - SYMPTOM DAILY DIARY 2013

14 January 2013

It's a new year and I survived the year of 2012, I never thought I would have made it but I did. At the beginning, no one knew how my body would respond to the treatment. All anyone could do was to guess, but it was an educated and calculated guess that we took as regards the abiraterone drug within the Stampede drug trials programme. The year was an emotionally charged one, which sent my emotions haywire! Mine went thru like a male menopause! Hot flashes, sweats, mood swings, all really intense. But for all of this I now have an almost non-existent PSA level, but it was a challenge emotionally for all of us. Clearly I am very sensitive to this type of chemotherapy drug (abiraterone) and medically it has worked for me. All my usual drugs were taken this morning.

The snow is falling as I make my notes and it looks pretty outside, central heating is on inside and it just makes it almost perfect to be warm and alive. Having now transferred my care from my local hospital to that of Mount Vernon Hospital, I feel so much more at ease. The care I received from my local hospital in 2012, was on a whole good though, towards the end of 2012, I felt that my care was being placed into the hands of a specialist registrar that I did not have faith in nor did my partner, so much so that we lodged an official complaint.

I do feel at times those responsible for your care lose the plot. Care – Attention – Advice are all 24/7, anything short of these are unacceptable for a cancer patient, as our pains and issues are daily. Actually for any person requiring medical attention the same must be said. To have lodged a complaint in my condition only added additional stress on me, which I really could have done without, but it had to be done. Sometimes you have to speak up for those that are afraid to or don't know how to.

At the start of my treatment my PSA level was over 500ng/ml by the end of 2012 it had come down to a remarkable 0.05ng/ml, clearly I had endured a journey of pain, anguish, stress and uncertainty of life. As stated, my care was good, but during the last few months of 2012 a particular doctor assigned to the oncology department was tasked with my care and from day one I felt that we did not hit it off well, nor my partner.

On the three occasions we were seen by him, we felt that on none of these occasions were my fears and concerns competently answered by this doctor, to my and my partner's satisfaction, and nor were we ever made to feel comfortable in his midst.

English certainly was not his first language, that he had a good command of which, complicated matters further. Yes, my treatments were improving on one side of the coin, but on the flip side an undercurrent of concerns were floating to the top. Our English language when spoken orally and grammatically written is a wonderful thing. But the consultant took it upon himself to savage the language to my dismay. Insensitive to say the least, when you confuse the word disease with decease. Nothing short of a lack of professionalism and attention when you say, "I think we will continue the treatment," and, "since last time, we noted that he was polyuric and polydipsic and his blood sugar was found to be high and thankfully enough, you actually prescribed for him some metformin, which controlled his blood sugar beautifully." And if I am to be fair the incompetence lay also at the hospital administration unit that dictated the letter sent out to me and my GP.

Both statements were worded in a letter to my GP as regards updating my current medical situation. The complaint letter reply that came back to me read, "I was sincerely sorry to learn that the word 'decease' was used rather than 'disease' in the letter. This is an extremely regrettable error and an insensitive error for which I apologise wholeheartedly." I could go on but I won't as in the end matters were resolved by carrying out the complaint, but also transferring my care to another hospital that was ranked in the UK's top five cancer centres. So a new chapter started to as regards my cancer care and I firmly believed it would benefit me in the long run.

My relationship with Grace and my children was now at an unbelievable all time high. I felt nurtured, loved and surrounded by so much genuine empathy. There were many times during 2012, that I felt that Grace and my personal relationship would not survive or continue, but it did and for that, I give thanks to the almighty. As I approached my 55th birthday in March, I did so with a certain amount of reservation, as this was the age my mother Hermelita Elvie Samuels died from her long battle with cancer. So a certain amount of apprehension existed for me as the clock turned back thirty years come March 2103, as I recollected her journey. For a period of seven years, she suffered with breast and lung cancer before succumbing.

My mother only asked two things during her illness, Firstly – that God allowed her to see her children grow up and secondly – That we her older children look after the younger ones our siblings. To be quite honest that has transpired and I am very happy to have been a part of the second request. My fight against cancer is largely a mirror of seeing her fight the same disease. My faith is seeing her accept fully the lord Jesus Christ into her life. She was a loving, caring, thoughtful mother, much of these traits which I find in Grace.

I am totally devoted to Grace and her to me. I know this because I see it in her eyes, as well as in her heart and it is said the "eyes are the windows to the soul". The scripture says "Luke 11:34: The lamp of the body is your eye. When your eye is simple, your whole body is also bright; but when it is wicked, your body is also dark." Thus, my understanding is that the eyes and heart are in alignment with each other.

I feel that resting on my shoulders the weight of a taboo that has plagued this family and it's up to me to not just try, but to break it. At the offset of my treatment, I never thought I would be able to continuously and regimentally take prescribed medication but I have and continue to each day, 5 tablets on an empty stomach before breakfast, 1 hour later 6 tablets with breakfast and 6 tablets just before bedtime. This has been my life for almost 11 months, without hesitation, without question like a soldier obeying an order from an officer I take my life saving medication.

I see now that I have a fighting chance to beat this disease and as such now is the time to finally settle down with Grace based on this reasoning. In the midst of my cancer suffering, I often remind myself Grace actually was more than a light that God sent me. When he placed her in my life, he placed an angel, rest assured there were others around, but not placed. It was for me to see through all the pretence and camouflage and choose richness and goodness that was and is to be. I have decided that when the time is right the proposal will be made and it will be the best proposal and occasion for *popping* the question; the future is bright and good for us.

Social economic problems are before us all and I have had my fair share of these, but what concerns me now is my ultimate happiness, everything else is secondary. I am without a doubt blessed and to be honest and open with you, I always thought that I was special. As I raise my head from my notebook, I can see the rooftops and tree lines are peppered with snow white and we are having a traditional post-Christmas scenery. It's so lovely looking out through my window today and feeling the way I do.

Lord, I ask, may I have more time please, so as to put the wrongs right? Many people do not get this chance in their life, but I know I am blessed to be able to do so and have done so and for that I am eternally grateful. As we wander through life we at times forget that there are consequences for everything that we do, equally we put off many important and not so important things for another day. Some of us never manage to see that "another day" some of us do, but are incapacitated from doing anything about it and just vegetate out.

God has a plan for me, in fact, he has a plan for us all. I do not know what mine is in his eyes, but I do know that his time differs greatly to my time. I am hoping that I have time on my side to finish my book, so that it will hopefully have an impact on many who will suffer and walk the cancer pathway. When you put things off remember that illness and death do not and will not wait, and can come to you at anyplace, anywhere or anytime.

22 January 2013

Well, today is a consultation day at the new hospital Mount Vernon. I came here yesterday on the 21st of January, for my bloods and today I am attending to get my new PSA level results. I am feeling apprehensive since yesterday, as is Grace. It's funny, I can always sense her apprehension, as her mood becomes sullen as opposed to me who just becomes quieter and reflective. The weather today was very cold with snow and ice covering the roads, but I didn't really feel it as such. I looked at myself in the mirror this morning and talked to myself, 'Al you're looking good, looking real good'. Usually when I'm sick, it clearly shows in my face, but not over the past few weeks and today I felt very well in myself.

Over the past few weeks I've gotten into light physical exercise again, ten minutes of hard physical exercise each day and the results were showing as my blood pressure was now down to 125/75. Having booked an appointment at my GP today he confirmed that my blood pressure was at the top end of the normal range it's virtually one year since my diagnosis and I have to say it's been an epic roller coaster of a journey. There is a saying that goes "unless you've walked a mile in these shoes, then you have no idea what one has gone through." Nothing has changed as I still endure much pain, anguish, loss of libido and heartache to mention but a few.

159

In all that I have gone through my family has been a tower of strength to me, especially my partner. A true fighter is what many have called me, personally I say a gladiator. You are what you do, not what you say. My entire lifestyle has changed to a more balanced lifestyle and continues to be so. There is no quick fix for cancer and neither is it for the faint hearted, cancer may be a curse, but with all curses, there are magical spells to counter. Cancer is only consistent with its meaning, not in how each and every one of us undergoes and deals with it, because it affects us all differently. The pain threshold of one person is very different to that of the next man or woman, boy or girl.

This disease has eaten away at my body and mind; it has tortured my spirit and taken me beyond a pain tolerance level even after using morphine. There was no such thing as a bad day just another day. Another day of feeling the aches, pains and fatigue in my bones and the seemingly never-ending dark depths of darkness.

Countless times the desire to give up and stop taking my medication preyed on my mind. But to give up was never ever in my character, it was not me; it was neither in my vocabulary nor my demeanour. Today, as I sat in the waiting room at Mount Vernon Hospital, surrounded by other cancer sufferers and listening to snippets of their woes and more woes, I knew that I was very, very, lucky indeed to still be alive. You could see in people's faces and hear how the disease has not only eaten away at them physically but also mentally, but also their desire to live any longer was no longer there.

Call it a sixth sense, that subtle perception that one has at times, but it was there written in their faces. Grace sat next to me whilst I made some notes for the diary unaware of the notes I was making as she was engrossed in reading from her Kindle. She seemed far more relaxed than earlier, though I felt in the air her apprehension as we waited, but she smiled through it and that comforted me. Hospitals are not a place you usually go to get smiles and all around us smiles were lacking.

I reflected last night on my life yet again, concluding that I had lived a fairly clean and balanced life, never taking anything in return for what I had done for others, always showing a kind and generous personality. I always believed that if it came it came, but I did not ever go looking for it.

My reflections on my life have lead me in all directions of late, the past, the present and the future had been dissected and minutely examined, even the future got an uncanny look in. I felt at times I had unknowingly been given an insight into this aspect already, through moments of relapse. I am held together by an iron will and determination that cancer will not and cannot break. Even though at times I am crying and hurting, I know eventually that I will be stronger and healthier, as I'm adamant that I am not going to let the cancer control my life, as it had tried to do on so many occasions.

My heart beats a healthier and stronger beat every day, as I put away my worries and strife. I feel that I can run to the end of the earth and back and I will survive and move forward and not look back, for there won't be anything gaining on me anymore, because I will have been cured. My appointment time came and I was summoned into the consultation room and my oncology care team were introduced to me.

After all introductions and pleasantries were exhausted, we got down to the reason for my transfer to Mount Vernon, which we revealed. With the air cleared now and the direction of my medical care direction discussed, my new PSA result was revealed. A reading of less than 0.1 was recorded which, at first we thought was an actual increase as the last reading recorded was 0.05.

However, it was explained that Mount Vernon hospital only gives readings down to the minimum level; of 0.1 in other words the reading could have been similar to the previously recorded result or lower. Therefore, once again, my PSA level remained low and from here on in virtually undetectable would be how it would be recorded. The

New Year had started so well and the glancing look Grace and I gave to each other said it all - The Cancer was well under control.

26 January 2013

The world today is one year to the day since I was officially diagnosed with prostate cancer. I am still alive, kicking and smiling plus holding onto a positive attitude.

It's been a hard slog and a painful one also, but now I have overcome this part of the journey. I have mixed feelings though to be quite honest, my medication has caused me at times to feel like I am moving from a state of clarity to a state of confusion and pain and visa versa. During these highly charged emotional times I realised that there were many people like me fighting to survive cancer. I also realised that the 'C' word was everywhere. Cancer to me is now just a word not a sentence, some people think that to be strong is to never feel pain in reality; the strongest people are the ones who feel it, understand it, and accept it. Spiritually, I don't believe God brought me this far to leave me dangling and alone. Though my tears have been plenty this storm is my test, it won't be long I just have to hold on a little longer.

We are now 15 months after the start of my cancer treatment programme today is June 27, 2013 and I am still very much alive and kicking. The treatment is going very well and my PSA level remains under a constant reading of less than 0.1. Only occasionally do I feel some pain that reminds me of my illness. Physically and mentally I am in a stronger place, some people think that to be strong is to never feel pain, but in reality, the strongest people are the ones who feel it, understand it, and accept it. My oncologist recently mentioned that it is a miracle what has happened to me; nothing short of a miracle. I cannot thank the Lord enough for walking with me through this painful, stressful, and emotional time as well as my family.

I have wondered at times if certain friends, family, and colleagues have really understood my cancer journey - they say they did, but on numerous occasions, they showed an unmindful, unperturbed, and pitiless attitude to their characters that was far from human behaviour. Sometimes in the solitude of the night I would shed a few tears, and find myself in moments of emotional imbalance as my thoughts rested on those people. Then it dawned on me that those things were adding to the emotional roller coaster, the stress, and the pain. Therefore, I opted for the positivity in my character, as opposed to the negativity, it then followed that positive thinking allowed me to do everything better than negative thinking did.

Cancer has still left me with no desire to love intimately. It has ripped the soul out of my heart, leaving me in emotional turmoil as the hormone injection is pumped into my body with purposeful effect. It regularly questioned my partner and me as to our loyalty to one another and in remaining in a relationship. When the intelligent head was in full swing, it said no matter how bad it is someone, somewhere was having it far worse than we were.

Almost daily around me were constant cancer reminders in the form of TV ads, radio show broadcasts, newspaper articles, leaflets all playing to my already battered set of emotions. My head is bowed as I review and mull over the past 18 months and I can only conclude that without a doubt, I am one lucky bloody fellow indeed. I have been given a second chance; I repeat a second chance, which many people do not get. Using it wisely, is the best advice I can give myself, for we rarely in life get a second chance. It is better to see everything from a positive perspective, so that the mind and heart are open to all possibilities, "for nothing will be impossible with God."

Today I met the football club manager for league two club, Bury FC, Kevin Blackwood, as my son Nathan, who is a professional footballer, was headhunted by this club and my son along with myself were invited to visit the club, with a view to potentially signing him. For me it was a rather long journey, having to travel from home to Euston station and then departing from British rail Euston into Manchester

Piccadilly and then a cab to the club's ground in Bury. As my son resided in Birmingham, we opted to meet in Birmingham and travel up from there together. When we arrived at the club, we were immediately introduced to Kevin and subsequently the management team and club chairman. I actually took to Kevin immediately and found him to be a plain straight-talking man with a knowledge and thirst for football. As we talked further, it became clearer why he and I gelled so well. Unfortunately, his daughter was yet another candidate for the "Lots of people fighting to survive cancer group" as she was suffering with cancer and in his words, "had been to hell and back."

My admission that I had cancer fell on sympathetic and caring ears, hence the connection. Today though I was there to support and advise my son, who himself was going through a bit of a roller coaster in life. His dad had cancer and his football career was not progressing as well as it could be, and here was a chance for him to get back up onto the football ladder rung, by dusting himself off, and moving onwards and upwards with a little advice and direction from me. He had the skills, strength, desire, psyche and they were interested in him. As I said earlier in this book, a parent's role never stops, not even for cancer. We must always lead by example, even in illness; children look to us no matter what.

Having toured the club grounds and discussed in depth the deal on offer, I felt that this was a good club for him to be at, if only short term, as he headed back up to at least championship level, where his career commenced. After a brief discussion with my sons' agent and my son himself, he happily agreed and signed to join the club as a first team player. I felt that the career of my son was now in firm hands. Life is so funny with the twists and turns. Cancer affects so many people. It's so unfair to see the damage that it causes.

In talking with Kevin Blackwell, I found that my emotional state was tweaked and again I felt that I had not gotten over, talking about it to anyone and maybe I'll never get over it. To date we still have not found the cure for this dreaded disease. How many more families have to be torn apart by this traumatic disease. As I sat there and drifted back in thoughts, I am truly amazed at what I had experienced and been through. God only knows how much, he will allow you to endure, for he is a truly wonderful God.

We departed the club and made our way back to the station, for our train journey back south. On our journey back, I took the liberty of speaking with him at length as regards keeping an eye and checking on his prostate on a regular basis. Obviously due to the family history as regards cancer this was a no brainier. I arrived home close to midnight and my mind and body were completely frazzled and fatigued, so to bed immediately I went.

Chapter 6 - SYMPTOM DAILY DIARY 2014

15 July 2014

I awoke today feeling apprehensive, as over the past two weeks I had been feeling rather unwell. The pains in my legs have returned, causing me to wince often during the daytime and occasionally during the night. Though, on one particular occasion the pain remained constant, for between three to four hours. This caused me to take 1.5 ml of oramorph breakthrough medication, something that I rarely have had to do. During the worst period of the pain, the left side of my head ached painfully causing me to clutch my head. My chest and stomach felt tender and painful. My lower back and upper shoulder, left and occasionally right sides ached with stabbing pains. My left and right hip joints were also painful. It felt at times that I had been cursed with the "variety-pack", of never knowing what would hit, where it would hit, where it would attack me, how long it would last, or the intensity of the pain. If I could only trade, my pains, but what would I trade them for, was the elusive question.

All I just wanted was my life back, to almost how it was prior, but things had changed forever and I had to learn to live with it. Had a consultation appointment with Mount Vernon Hospital as my GP had written a letter to the Oncologists' Department requesting that an MRI scan be carried out, to see what the state of my bones were. A considerable amount of time had passed, since I had last been scanned, so I was somewhat apprehensive which was further compounded, by the need to know what my new PSA reading results were.

Grace took the day off work to attend, as she had witnessed all the pains that I had been subjected to and could support my version of events, far more accurately. She has been through a lot these past few weeks, besides her own medical ailments she has watched me writhe in pain, on numerous occasions. The real worry for us both though we don't discuss it verbally, is a concern that my PSA level may have risen. This could account for the reason why my pains had returned. Clutching at straws and stabbing in the dark, was what we had been doing over the past few weeks, as to what it could be or not be.

We arrived on time, sat in the waiting room, and waited for our appointment. The usual procedure carried out when I attend the clinic is that I check in at reception and then I am directed to the waiting room, to wait for the research nurse who usually presents herself in person and leads us to her office. Questions are then asked about my health since the last consultation, after which my PSA results are revealed to me. This is then followed up with my blood pressure being taken and recorded and my next appointment arranged.

I am then seen by the oncologist or registrar to ensure all the right ticks are in the boxes, to keep the trials programme committee happy and answer any questions that we may have. He then officially signs off on my new script, namely the abiraterone and prednisolone medication tablets for the next month of treatment. After all this was completed, I was good to leave the hospital and go home. The whole process usually takes about one hour from arrival to finish.

Today, however, was different as we arrived at the hospital and waited in the line at reception to report in. I felt a soft tap on my shoulder and turned to see in front of me a very old school friend of mine, who had been referred to the Hospital by his GP with a raised PSA level of 17, which had just dropped to 14. This I knew because during the weeks previous he had telephoned me complaining that he was not happy with the cancer team dealing with his care, so I suggested that he got his doctor to refer him to my hospital for a second opinion which, clearly he had done. His wife accompanied him, and we all greeted each other. As I looked into his face I saw a gaunt person, who to me looked a fraction of his former self. He had always been a guy with a slim stature, on this occasion he looked very different. I was glad to see him, but was concerned at what I was seeing.

After a few words, we parted ways, as he had his appointment to attend, and I mine. Today was an unusually busy day at the hospital. Due to the contents of my GP's letter, it was deemed necessary that I undergo an MRI scan once again. The scan would take approximately twenty minutes, and gave an update on the state of my bones and my back. I changed into the provided gown and entered into the MRI scan room. Having had MRI scans in the past, I felt that there was nothing unduly to concern myself about.

Little did I know what lay ahead. I was summoned into the X-ray room and lay on my back on a flat bed conveyor unit, which would electronically pull me into a large tubular type chamber unit, whereupon the scanning process would commence. Headphones were to be placed over my head with selected music playing. I was asked if I was comfortable and I said yes and the described process commenced. I felt the flat bed conveyor pulling me into the tubular chamber, but as my body partially reached inside the unit a feeling of claustrophobia came over me, I shouted out, "Get me out of here! Get me out of here!" to which I was returned to the comfort of normality.

I immediately sat up and the buzzing question on my mind was why I was freaking out? This was not me; I had done this scan on three previous occasions. What was so different now? The radiologist asked me if I was all right and I nodded yes and then said to her, "There's no way I could do this, sorry." She replied by saying that she was a little concerned prior to me entering the unit as she felt I might not fit comfortably into the unit.

I returned to the changing room, changed, and then returned to Grace in the waiting room who was surprised to see me back so quick. I explained to her what had occurred as she looked at me in amazement. I was returned to the research nurse who used a tape measure to measure the circumference of my waist. It was only at this moment when I realised what had happened, it had been 2 years since the last scan and at that time, I was weighing around 121kg. However, my weight since then had increased and I was now a bulky 134kg. This was the reason why and it was scary. Real scary.

Well, fortunately for me a larger machine was available, and an hour later I was placed on this unit and pulled through and the sensation of claustrophobia was a remote distance. Though, I was not to get away unscathed again, the hot flushes just decided to play havoc and as I lay there the sweat poured off my face. I recall just shutting my eyes and saying to myself, "You have to grin and bear this, it is important that they are able to scan the body just a few minutes and you'll be fine."

The machine was very noisy and looked archaic. The scan finished and the radiologist entered the room and came to where my head lay. I recall her saying, "Look at the sweat pouring off you. Are you ok?"

I nodded and she pressed the button to pull me back to the safety of air. With that, the scan was completed, but it meant now that future scans using MRI was out of the question for me, but I was not complaining, not at all.

I recall my army days of combat training in our unit where a test for claustrophobia was for soldiers to be subjected to underground tunnel training. A team of four would enter at one point in an underground tunnel system with just enough space to enter/exit and to be able to crawl on all fours or belly crawl if you so wished, and be required to find their way out at a given exit point. Having a man's bottom in your face was no joke, especially in the depths of darkness and limited air. Working as a team, we passed that phase of our training. Now many years later I could not even pass through a medical scan machine a further feeling of incapability.

15 August 2014

These past few days I have felt that I have just been going through the motions. I have felt very unsteady on my feet, my sense of balance has not been completely there, and I found at times through the day that I just staggered around the house bumping into furniture and things. The sweating was still very apparent with most mornings sweat imprints visible on my pillow. I met with Celena today as I had promised her that I would accompany her to see an herbal specialist, in West Wickham, Surrey whom she uses and has a high regard for. As I drove to meet her thoughts were running through my mind as to whether this was a good idea or not. Though, it must be said that two of my sisters use her services also, so three people couldn't be wrong I thought. On arrival, pleasantries were exchanged and I had a one-to-one consultation with her and acknowledged my illness to her. I found her easy to converse with and empathetic, as well as knowledgeable about my illness. This consultation was long overdue, as I had promised to attend with Celena many months ago, but one thing leading to another I never made it.

Nothing before its time I say because, as we travelled back to home, out of the blue a conversation struck up between us and certain revelations came out.

"Dad," she said, "you have to get to grips with the sweating issues you are undergoing as it affects the relationship with your children.

It has been over two years now and we your children cannot plan to do anything much with you, due to having to always consider if a particular environment is suitable for you to be physically in. Many a time we have wanted to take you out to restaurants, but were unable to do so because we knew you would be very uncomfortable and conscious of your sweating episodes as and when they came on."

"We don't care about your sweating dad and rest assured no one is looking at you when you have these episodes. Also, we find that we cannot travel with you, in your vehicle as when we do, you have the air conditioning fully up to compensate for your sweating and we get extremely cold, but do not want to say anything to cause you to become upset."

A tear came to my eye as we drove, and then a few more and I found I was unable to drive for a moment, as my vision became impaired. My daughter realised the impact this conversation had and my reaction and immediately changed the subject which, personally I was happy for.

I had not forgotten all that had been said and yes, I have been always very conscious that when I sweated profusely that people in our midst might be looking and wondering, "What's the matter with this guy?" Obviously unbeknownst to them I am a cancer patient suffering from the side-effect of the prostap hormone injection. On numerous occasions prior to my cancer diagnosis I had reflected on how well I was personally doing in life in general. I could so easily have carried on in life without the knowledge that I had prostate cancer, despite it being the most common cancer diagnosis among men in the UK. I would have just carried on with daily life, oblivious to the underlying danger and then it would have been far too late for me. So I suppose my children are correct, a little sweat here and there was nothing to concern myself about at all as I so often had done.

September 30, 2014

I awoke feeling somewhat lethargic and fatigued but had no real pain to complain about which has been the case now for many months. Today I attended an early morning appointment with the Mount Vernon Hospital care team to review my latest PSA blood results which were taken yesterday. I attended my hospital appointment for the first time unaccompanied, as Grace had just started a new job and could not afford the time off, to attend with me.

It felt very strange in fact eerie, she was always there in attendance, my rock, my pillar, my confidant. It felt like my right hand was adrift, severed. It became very apparent when I entered the building and saw other patients with their husbands, wives, partners, family members, or otherwise. Hospitals are daunting places at the best of times, but a cancer centre treatment hospital is a far more depressing establishment to attend by yourself and I personally would always advise against it if at all possible.

We as humans are psychosomatic by nature. Our well-being is greatly influenced by our behaviour, emotions, thoughts, and social interaction. If we wish to care for our well-being, we must care for our lifestyle, our mental, emotional, and interactive world. When we have nice experiences, then we are happy. Take away those nice experiences, then we become fearful. In other words, with family and friends around to support in whatever way, we are relatively happy regardless of the dilemma we are facing. With no one there to be supportive, we instinctively become fearful, of our surroundings.

Those charged or responsible for our care do not necessarily see the best in or from us. Have you ever wondered why our blood pressure readings differ, sometimes vastly when we are at our doctors or a hospital environment as opposed to being at home? The fear in sickness connected to the fear of dying is the greatest fear that we as human beings have. We have no idea what will happen to us after we die as such, we are therefore afraid of the unknown. As I have said this is my personal take on it, after three years of toing and froing medical facilities and establishments.

Arrived as usual with punctuality and checked in at reception. The clinic did not seem that busy and was unusually quiet. A short while after being seated the nurse presented herself to me and we walked to her office for our usual medical rap. I always found it nice to exchange pleasantries, as well as an informal chit-chat, as it allowed my mind to be taken away from the current environment. Adults are not afforded the same distractions and attractions that are offered to children who are able to interact with and focus on images on the wall, which help with distraction during procedures and appointments. All we see is nothing but cancer -related information in one sense or another. Oh, to be a child again. My blood pressure was taken resulting in a reading of 148/78 with a pulse of 70, ear temperature taken result normal, weight today 132.7kg. I recalled raising my eyebrows, as it seemed to have increased which surprised me especially, as I had been working out physically recently.

The quarterly clinical trials unit quality of life form, was thrust before me to complete again. This is a list of questions that are set out before me to complete, by encircling questions such as do you have any trouble doing strenuous activities - like carrying a heavy shopping bag or suitcase or do you have problems with long or short walks or the more invasive questions such as to what extent were you interested in sex over the past four weeks.

I can see the point where some of these questions are leading, as I undergo a few of these issues at times. But, I do not want to always answer at times, especially the invasive questions as you do feel that your manliness is being questioned by these composites of the qualities of being human. After finishing the questionnaire, I ventured along to see the senior oncologist, as I had expressed a desire to see him, as I was going away on holiday and it seemed very appropriate to do so. The doctor was quick to pass on my PSA results, which once again were less than 0.1, and in his words "undetectable," a word that I had become so familiar with.

Within me, a sense of emotional fulfilment was going on, as I focused on that word "Undetectable."

What followed next was for the first time ever in my treatment an evaluation of where they believed I stood medically. I asked the doctor where he saw things going for me forthwith. And I quote: -

"Alfred, without a doubt yours is a miracle cure to date; we have a number of people on this trial that are 2 yrs plus into the programme that have responded like you have. We also have a few people who have been on the programme for 5 yrs and are still responding favourably. Even if your PSA were to rise above the concern level, we have in our armoury other medications that we can use to control the rise."

You can imagine the elated feeling that that statement gave me. Those words uttered gave me a further sense of upliftment as well, as if had I taken a happy pill to place me in that feel-good factor realm. Today was definitely one of the better clinic visits that I had attended.

We shook hands as I departed his office and recalled passing the waiting room where other patients were waiting to see the oncologists, with a smile on my face. In fact more like a smirk hoping that not only would they have good news, but that they could see and feel my joy and excitement as I continued "Coming out the other side."

I left the building and headed to my car where I sent a number of texts to my nearest and dearest.

There were times that I had considered asking Grace to give her account of what she had gone through and experienced with me. But it became clear that there were a number of things that she wanted to keep private between us and not for publication and some of which I also will never be privy to "that special place where we all store special memories and moments."

Chapter 7 - MESSAGES OF SUPPORT

Texting makes the lines of communication a wondrous thing. I look back at many a text message received from family and friends and still a tear rolls down my cheek.

27.01.12 Grace my partner at 0:58 hours

"The last six months has been one of the happiest times in my life for a long time because you have been part of it and will continue to be, whatever is ahead I will be with you every step of the way

02.02.12 Kelly my brother at 16:26 hours

You are a terrific Bro keep strong.

14.02.12 Celena my daughter at 20:44 hours

It's only natural to feel that way, hopefully the pain will ease off and allow you to do a bit at a time. Only do what you can whatever you can't do you just leave it. Don't let the cancer take over the fight hasn't even begun yet.

14.02.12 Celena my daughter at 20:58 hours

Remember, you said this was going to be a long road; it's of course going to take its toll on you worse when the pain hits you. xxx

02.03.12 Lajade my daughter at 14:32 hours

Ha ha, yeah no tears. Just have to be a fighter just like my daddy.

03.03.12 Valentina my sister at 18:10 hours

Just remember your heavenly father loves you and is watching over you, you are never alone. Standing in the gap in prayer for you. God is not finished with you yet, big brother. By the way, thanks for being my big brother should have told you years ago love you.

05.04.12 Kira my daughter @ 12.05 hours

"Hi, I'm sorry for the late reply just got credit on my phone I didn't want to bother you with how I feel I just need time and I'm just finding it really hard, however, I'm here for you 1000% and positive thinking equals positive outcomes ....Love You xxx".

25.04.12 Valentina my sister @ 18.50 hours

Valentina texts me it reads "Just remember he neither sleeps nor slumbers, he continues to watch over you even when others have gone. His faithfulness is everlasting to all who call upon him".

26.04.12 Grace my partner @ 08.42 hours

"I feel we have got so much closer over the past few months and share something special. I need you to know I am here for you and my love for you grows ever.

10.06.12 Grace my partner 12:33 hours

Sometimes I do not know what to do for the best, but I want you to know I am always here for you, and I love you with all my heart. G xxxx

18.07.12 Kira my daughter at 22:36 hours

You're a soldier.

20.07.12 Grace my partner at 08:10 hours

It has been a wonderful 1st year and I'm looking forward to many more wonderful years xxx G

21.07.12 Celena my daughter at 11:41 hours

Not sad, that's what the fight is all about for this draining cancer unfortunately dad.

13.08.12 Kira my daughter at 21:00 hours

Thank you dad! I'm so glad I have seen you. You're looking well xxx

06.09.12 Grace my partner at 11:58 hours

Yet let's you always think you will, those important to you I headed yourself, that's why you are so special and one of the many things I love about you...xxx

12.09.12 Nathan my son at 16:23 hours (replying to a text that I had sent out about my PSA results dropping)

Brilliant news dad very, very, happy

12.09.12 Lajade my daughter at 16:24 hours

Yaaayyy lol smiles and grins with you. Mummy said that's good.

13.09.12 Valentina my sister at 11:19 hours

What do you mean maybe? We are fighters remember that till the very last breath

09.10.12 Celena my daughter at 19:51 hours

As you know nobody said it was going to be a breeze or easy, each day as it comes.

25.10.12 Nathan my son at 00:08 hours (replying to a text I had sent out about PSA results dropping)

Yes, Dad such great news so pleased very happy so proud of you for fighting so hard and keep on fighting

Best Friend Tosin Bex-Banjo – Inscribed on the inside of a book gift to me

To: Alfi
Respect to you as a warrior I know you'll win this fight.
29 December 2012

September 30, 2014 12.10 hours

Received text from Grace which said the following "And we keep marching on, fighting this thing they call cancer - every day I see your battle and every day I pray you keep fighting to go on, words cannot express how I feel to see you climbing those hills (she is referring to my outdoor fitness training activity) even when you think you cannot do one more hill you do, that is my inspiration to carry on also to.

That fighting spirit will keep you here not for five but for the next 10 years plus... you heard what the doctor said this morning as he referred to the small group; well you were placed on this arm of the stampede drug trial programme by God. He knew what he was doing when he placed you there. He was not ready for you then and is still not ready for you now as he knows just like I do you have so much still left to do and so many more lives yet still to touch."

Text from my son James Dec 8th, 2014 @ 11.29am...

Remember Dad your sons are watching and learning how to behave in the face of any of our future adversities soldering on staying strong...

Text from an old school friend Jan 12th, 2015 @ 10.43am
Prostate Cancer Patient)

Alf, I hope and pray that all goes well for you. You have been a tower of strength for me and I appreciate that. God bless and here's wishing you well. Hughie

Chapter 8 - TWO YEARS DOWN THE LINE

Here I am, two years down the line, reflecting back on so much. I cannot believe that two years have passed so quickly and I am still alive, as well as responding incredibly to the treatment. It was only yesterday that my thoughts bordered on a society where the "so called powerful" mandated that they cut, eradicate, medicate, "chemo ate", at peoples bodies. There was in my mind a danger that this became the normal acceptance, that this was the best and/or only treatment for cancer. I had often wondered what about prevention and alternative and complimentary therapies.

The internet is great but you can't believe everything you read online especially unproven nonsense about miracle cancer cures. Nowadays people are far more sceptical as to what they believe in. I think many people including myself believe there is a cure out there, but the pharmaceutical industry chooses not to pursue it because they are making so much money in another direction.

My recent belief is now, quality of life over quantity. I would rather have one month of real life than a lifetime stuck in a hospital, unable to do the things I love. It would be one thing if I thought the treatment would mean I would eventually be able to return to my life, but not if the treatment and hospitals would "be" my life. But that was while I was in a confused state of mind, as well as a selfish state of mind.

What about my children? What about my new soul partner whose personality, beauty and compassion I had been searching for many years to make myself totally whole? I'm currently on a roller coaster that can only go up.

After many months of treatment, I began to realise that the hormone therapy treatment Prostap had impaired my thinking and mental function. This had persisted for two years leaving me with fuzzy mental functioning along with fatigue and bouts of depression. This compounded with the negative thoughts I was having, was becoming destructive to my health. The constant idea that something might happen was banging away in my head, leading me into dark regions of anxiety and fear. If you have bad thoughts and bad feelings, you are going to have a bad reaction, and this is what happened, culminating in me feeling sicker and sicker at times.

My business partners meant me well in general, but business must continue and at times, my absence and lack of mental input caused major issues.

I lost a great deal of money during the first year of my illness, along with a bit more during the second, but as the late reggae singer Bob Marley said, "Money is numbers and numbers never end. If it takes money to be happy, your search for happiness will never end." I found that I was allowing this to swallow me up, as well as trying to stay well. Trust me, both decisions don't walk in harmony.

I have worked hard all of my life and never, ever envisaged, that cancer would strike me down and make me so ill. Athletics, fitness, yoga and squash were all regular parts of my fitness regime, resulting in my visits to my doctor occurring only every five years after the age of twenty. One could suggest I surrounded myself with an air of invincibility and they would not be far from wrong. An athletics sprint champion competitor at county schools and British AAA levels for three *consecutive* years. A former member of an elite unit within the British Territorial Army and a top-class close protection officer to the entertainment, corporate industries for 28 years were just some of the experiences that best described my way and style of life.

The question of how cruel life could be nagged me when cancer struck. I suppose I misunderstood that illness and death waits for no one. It comes at the least expected moment without favour or prejudice. I had advanced metastatic prostate cancer. Why couldn't I have a lesser

181

curable type of cancer? I suppose because maybe the fight would not have been as hard as it was now. Why can't we find a cure for cancer after all these years and loss of life, of dear and close ones, why, why, why? I often wonder what life would have been like for the ones we lost so cruelly to cancer. My mother was only 55 years old when she succumbed to the disease. I recall my godmother telling me, in the talks that she had with my mother, that she would often say she prayed to God, to allow her to see her children grow up into young adults. This, he granted her; now, I am asking the same.

God allowed this; the youngest of us was 18 years old and the oldest 25 when she died. Sometimes, I think I am being prepared unknowingly for my appointment with the Almighty and the time I have left is to be used wisely. Many others don't get that second chance in life.

I was very close to my mother and made sure she did not want for anything before cancer took her from us. I hate the word 'cancer' with a passion; it took from me one of the world's best and greatest mothers and other family members, and was now here, trying to take me from my family and loved ones. Well, I have news for you, CANCER: I'm going to fight you just like my mother did. I'm going to give you one hell of a fight, hopefully leaving you so weak that you will be weakened and exhausted, and become incapable of causing me, your host body, any further harm.

I only wish I could go ten rounds with cancer in a boxing ring, as I am confident and sure that I would knock it clean into outer space. I am sure there are many out there who agree with me, as I know I am not the only one who has lost close ones to cancer. I would want to think that my positive side is keeping me away from the debilitating, depressing and destructive side of my fight against cancer. Of course, at times, nothing seems attractive to me and I do feel unmotivated to get out of these states. However, I have decided not to cling to depressing thoughts, and to instead try to tune into the positivity that is before me.

Sometimes negativity and weakness overwhelmed me to the point that, in order to get out of these states, I needed a 'bombardment of positivity' to get me out of that into which I allowed myself to be closed. Nobody can do it for you; you have to take the steps to place yourself in the right frame of mind to deal with cancer.

In saying this though, people say the strangest things to someone with cancer, if only people would take time out to understand and realise the impact, of some of the supportive comments. Typically for me a few were:-

How are you feeling? How the bloody hell do you think I'm feeling? I have cancer! How would you feel?! Next!

Have you tried praying? Really? Now is the time you want to proclaim your faith? I write this as a person who believes in the almighty: however, please keep your personal beliefs to yourself. Now is not the time for missionary work.

Think positive?

Is thinking positive and cultivating a happy and balanced outlook important to me with cancer? Absolutely. Is telling me to think positive even the slightest bit helpful? No, not at all.

You can beat this. You're strong!

I won't die of cancer because I've "lost the will to fight." That's an incredibly simplistic way of looking at it. People die of cancer because their tumour burden is simply too high and sometimes chemotherapy is ineffective depending on the type of cancer. This has nothing to do with the will to live, or one's personal character, or how much suffering I am experiencing.

You'll be fine

Are you my doctor. Are you just saying this because you want me to be fine but really know that no one knows how this is all going to play out? I hope so. I hope you face up to the reality that I did: that no one knows or has control over what happens in the course of any life-limiting disease. Pretending everything is going to be fine is ridiculous and may I add condescending.

In reality I know they care about me, so that makes them great in my eyes, as it means they are trying to reach out to me. What else can I ask for beyond them reaching out to me. I'm the last person to actually give family, friends and concerned parties a hard time over awkward but well-meaning phrases.

In the end to be honest, the most important thing to say to someone with cancer is anything at all. Because the truth in reality is that the isolation from cancer is sometimes the worst part of the disease. Remember there is a person behind the diagnosis, who once regularly laughed and loved.

I write from my heart when I say this that metastatic cancer overrides your worst fears of pain. It's unimaginable to describe this type of cancer pain when it reaches and touches the human bones. They say tooth pain borders on some of the worst pain a human can endure, war injuries excepted. As an adult, dealing with this pain is one thing. When I think about a child suffering a similar fate, tears fall from my eyes not only for that child, but also for their parents. To look dauntingly upon the twisted, contorted face of their child lying, dying in front of them must be a life changing experience. Personally in my professional capacity I witnessed such an action as this and it changed me forever.I recall the searing pain late at night in the first year of treatment after haven taken my painkillers, Ibuprofen and MST. The contorted look on my partner's face as she watched me virtually leap into the air with these highly-charged spasms that I would undergo as the pain affected my body.

If one is to believe that pain is merely weakness leaving the body, then

I am well on the way to a full recovery. Coupling this with the side effects of hot sweats emanating as a result of the prostap hormone injection, you understand the living hell I have lived among others. Everyone has a handful of wishes in life, be it a new home, a new car, a holiday cruise. I, as a cancer sufferer, have only one wish: to get better.

Once again, it's been a while since I've made notes and a lot has gone on over the past few months. Where do I start? About myself, usually, and the beginning of the last few months seems ideal. The reason for my decreasing notation has been more than just not feeling up to it, nor well enough, but also the recurring events that affected my daily life. My PSA continues to come down from 0.19ng/ml to 0.05mg/ml, an unthinkable reading in the early part of the year, that is now a reality.

God continues to answer my prayers as He does for all those that continue to pray to Him. I am still in some pain, though in my lower back area as well as my right upper thigh. The recent scans undertaken (bone and CT scan) showed differences, though. My bone scan showed a reduction in or a total removal of lymph nodes in most previous areas scanned. Barring my right hip, which shows the same size and shape from day one, a vast improvement has occurred. Strangely, though, the CT scan gives a slightly different version of events, but nothing about which to unduly concern myself at this moment in time.

Today I wrote a poem, one which I would like to share.

THIS HEAVY LOAD I BEAR

Sometimes, life felt so unfair. Many a time, I felt alone and thought that no one seemed to really care. Sometimes, I felt I was drowning in despair and there was no one there, and all my hopes had vanished into thin air. Then, a voice entered my head and said "Hang in there my son, I am with you until the end. Just keep those hopes alive, keep holding on, you'll see the dawn take one more step, just one small step, that will allow me to hang on in there a little longer."

I have felt how life is filled with so much pain, like everything I try to do seemed all in vain. I have felt so fatigued and weary, and not wanting to go on, feeling these aches and tiredness in my bones. Then again, that voice entered my head and said "Hang in there my son, reach down inside, find the strength, let it be your guide. When the road ahead is so rough, don't give up, dig deep inside. Find that courage in your heart, don't ever lose hope, nor the will to fight."

Many a time I asked was there a god above, many a time I asked where was his love and mercy during my time of suffering.

No sign was given, nor audible reply heard and I continued to wonder further would I ever mend, would this darkness never end, so many things, so hard to comprehend. I started to become fearful, I started to doubt, so much bitterness inside, all these feelings that I cannot cast aside. Then, like a twinkling star on a dark clear summer's night, I remembered that voice and the words aloft in my mind. Today, I raised my head to the sky and a tear came to my eye as I said to the Lord "Thank you Lord, I now know why, just one more breath of life and one more step then I'll take."
In taking one more step I realised that the hardest part of the struggle against cancer was losing my will and determination to survive and for sure it happens to all cancer patients. Within a few weeks of commencing the stampede drugs trials programme I was so out of it mentally that all I wanted to do was lie down and die... I kid you not.

But there came a moment in time when I re-addressed my whole attitude towards surviving and the treatment that I was being given. So I got mad, took off my invisible boxing gloves and bared my knuckles to cancer and became a survivor of prostate cancer.

I had now made it a personal thing. This wasn't some mindless, faceless disease. This was something trying to ruin and ultimately take me away from my loved ones and my life, and for every stumble I had, it had a laugh at my expense. THAT... was motivation.

And like that, I learned a valuable lesson that day. I realised that in order to win the war against cancer, you have to find and embrace something that motivates you.

My motivation now is to help others get back up when they've been knocked down, and I will even include myself in that category. Cancer knocked me off my feet more times than I care to remember but in doing so I was forced to remember a verse , "It's not how many times you get knocked down. It's how many times you get back up." who ever dreamt that one up sure was someone much smarter than me.

But at this stage in my life here and now love conquers all. I really mean that, because that's what I was lead to and found.

Growing up as a young man youth and anger had gotten me through, but what would get me through now, more than doctors or chemo or support from outside, is the love I have for my partner and children, no matter how many more times it comes and knocks me down. "I am going to keep getting up you can bet on that.

I can look at prostate cancer from a negative perspective, or focus on the fact that it's one of the most manageable and curable medical conditions that can be treated.

Chapter 9 - Thyroid Cancer

Today is December 9 2014, and I attended a hospital appointment, to get a thyroid issue examined after its development 18 months prior. My doctor deemed it unnecessary to do anything about the issue until it caused me any issues. During the last six months, an issue developed where my voice started to change from the dulcet tones to which everyone was accustomed. It transformed into a somewhat croaky voice, hardly audible at times. My partner Grace attended the appointment with me to see a registrar of the specialist ENT consultant. On the last visit, we raised the issue of the croakiness; this was dismissed as an enlarged goitre and nothing more sinister. As such, I was discharged for a year.

Today, we were back to delve into my voice, which was fading significantly. Our appointment was set for 09:10 hours, but it was 09:40 hours before we were seen; lateness once again seemed the norm for the clinic. Pleasantries were exchanged and we sat with the registrar to discuss the issue at hand, as my GP had written a letter. Grace sat and listened as I relayed what had been going on over the past six months: the gruff voice, the almost non-existent voice when vocally challenged in talking to people and the breathlessness. The doctor listened pensively as I recalled the moments after which he suggested that he would carry out an endoscopy procedure, as what I was suggesting bordered on a sinister medical issue as related to my voice. The procedure was carried out with a tube inserted through my nose, down into my throat. It was a rather irritable, uncomfortable, invasive feeling, but I managed while he examined the throat. Upon doing so, he was able to see that one of my vocal cords was not responding accordingly, "you seem to have a lazy vocal cord," in his words. Having finished the procedure, his blunt diagnosis was that the inactivity of the cord could be due to thyroid cancer.

Well, wham, here I was again, facing that word 'cancer,' but on this occasion, Grace sat with me. I immediately looked over at her and saw her distorted face and her eyes exploding into an avalanche of tears; this was far from what we expected or wanted to hear. As I sat there, my mind wandered back to my prostate cancer diagnosis and how I felt then. At that very moment in time, I was without feeling; the despondency I felt previous was also lacking. The news was not good, but I did not feel fearful other than the usual question, 'why me?'

I looked back at the doctor, then across to Grace, who by now was very upset. The doctor commented that it was not the end of the world, as thyroid cancer was very treatable. However, this statement did not console Grace one bit, as she recalled that a dear friend of hers had died from thyroid cancer.

At this point, I think the doctor realised that he needed support and indicated that he wished to consult with the consultant, leaving the room in a hurry. With only Grace and I in the room, she reverted to some familiar words: "What am I going to do without you?"

My whole emotional blanket was torn down at these words and tears filled my eyes. If I had any notion that the word 'cancer' would have been mentioned in this consultation, I would never have subjected Grace to attend it. Tears were not on the horizon for me, but my emotions were evident more to Grace than myself.

I held and stroked her hands, telling her that we would just have to deal with it, the same way we have dealt with everything else. There was undeniably a strength and loving presence in the room that day and, once again, I felt that holy presence. A few minutes passed and the registrar re-entered the room, this time with the consultant, who arrived straight at the point before the blink of an eye. As he sat there, he looked me straight in the eye and reiterated his colleague's diagnosis, with neither a blink nor the twitch of a facial muscle as he talked to me. Maybe once or twice, his attention span crossed to Grace, but that lasted merely seconds before he fixed his attention back onto me.

From here on out, I renamed him the 'the Ice Man,' only because he was emotionless, but most definitely a seasoned professional used to delivering diagnoses of a chronic nature. In the room that day, it was clearly the master leading the apprentice, but also an icy chill had swept through in the form of the consultant. But you know what? I appreciated it in the end; it was a plain, straight to the point, no bullshit nor pretence diagnosis, which worked for me. After all, it wasn't Grace that was directly suffering, it was me. I listened as he recommended that an operation would be required, as it could be thyroid cancer. Although it could have also just been the mass of the goitre resting against my vocal cord, this, he dismissed, as my voice loss suggested something far more sinister.

Clearly, the medical route of the worst scenario was being played out before me with the lesser, an option.

The pros and cons of the operation were firmly laid out to us. There were risks involved: a possible total loss of voice or a possible infection in the resulting wound. Nonetheless, an operation was required, after which a histology would be carried out of the thyroid.

Should this be proven cancerous, radiotherapy treatment would be needed after, and hopefully there it would end.

With a clear understanding of what was ahead for me, the paperwork process started again. Blood tests, thyroid function and a CT body scan from head to stomach would be required prior to the operation. Eight weeks was the time frame the consultant gave, though the usual waiting time was 16 weeks. Due to the possible severity of the diagnosis, urgency was placed on my operation. The option for a shorter notice operation if one became available was also given to me, which I agreed to take if possible. By now, Grace had composed herself again, and that tough bulldog mentality approach and look was again showing on her face, instilling ease in my mind. She retook the reins and was actively engaged and leading the dialogue and decision-making as I sat, listening and saying very little.

Grace was now in full control of her emotions; however, I had been in control of mine from the moment the dreaded word 'cancer' was mentioned. You see, I had reverted into my survivalist mode, as, once again, my whole life had changed in just a few seconds, featuring daily 'normality vs. extremity.' The normality was self-evident; however, the extremity verged on the testimony of traumatic realism, which was the delivery of the terrible news seeking to contaminate my mind again.

In reality, though, underneath all this armour, a chink was starting to appear, though only I knew it was there. How much more could I take, mentally and physically? The answer lay in my head from a proverb: "God is faithful, and he will not let you be tested beyond your strength, but with your testing he will also provide the way out so that you may be able to endure it" (1 Corinthians 10:13). If I am to look beyond my own self-centeredness to the pain and severe testing others endure in the world, then, in reality, I have had it easy. What of those who wake up hungry each day? What about the abused, the victims of racism? What about the people of the world in certain parts of the Middle East or Africa, who have known no other life than a daily existence of war and terror?

Or could it be that God is using me to provide a 'way out' for the hopeless? Could I in some way help others handle life as relates cancer illnesses? I do wonder sometimes.

As we departed the hospital and drove home, the mood in the car was pensive and very little was said. The mood, however, said it all: now it starts all over again, and 'the family has to be told.' Neither were items I looked forward to undertaking again.

I found that informing my family a second time around was not so daunting as on the first occasion, not so painful and heart wrenching. I personally telephoned each of my children and explained the situation to them, but strangely, there were no tears or hysteria on their parts, although they voiced much concern. I attempted to downplay it as much as I could; I discussed the proposed operation and possible treatment options available to me, along with the risks mentioned. They were now fully informed and I felt once again an ease in my mind having done so. No doubt they would once again carry out their own research in the interim, something I had become familiar with and admired of them.

Having accomplished all of this, I sat with my arms propped against my chin and pondered my future. Once again, I was facing an uncertain future. The familiar words echoed through my mind: cancer, why me again, how much more could and would I take? Would I go through all the ill feelings once again during any subsequent treatment? Damn you, cancer, damn you again.

Now, my family and I faced another cancer battle: that of Thyroid cancer. Information suggested that this was by far the better of the two cancers to have (not to say any cancer is worth having). For me, a drawback was that the location of my goitre was hidden from view of any scan and this posed an issue for the medical team involved in confirming for sure that it was thyroid cancer, other than the change of voice.

Christmas 2014 was fast approaching and the mood in my household was somewhat duller than usual. I was very unhappy, but still I had to show a side to all that I would fight anything placed before me. I still had to inform Mount Vernon Hospital about the new development; this was carried out during my consultation with them at an appointment just before Christmas. As usual, Grace attended and we informed the doctor and staff accordingly. Having been under their care for almost two years, a family-like environment existed and a genuine concern for my health was apparent as they gasped and grappled with the news. The doctor, consultant and research nurse all showed empathy and I was moved, as was my partner. As we sat in the consultation room, my doctor, who was not convinced by the diagnosis theory, decided to investigate further. He requested that the ENT medical team fax over the previous set of test results taken almost 18 months previous so he could review for himself the validity of the diagnosis.

Now, I have to say, elation shuddered through my body at the thought of an incorrect diagnosis. I caught sight of Grace's face, which beamed like the Cheshire Cat that the possibility of this could be so true. The doctor made the call to the hospital and requested the fax be sent while I continued my usual tests. My PSA reading was once again less than 0.1ng/ml and all other blood function tests indicated that all was internally fine with me. As we were setting to leave the hospital, we received a telephone call from my doctor requesting that we visit his office. We did so; upon arriving, we were greeted by a document in his hand containing the results going back eighteen months ago, which stated categorically no sign of anything benign.

The possibility that I did not have thyroid cancer loomed in front of us. Did they get it wrong? The urge to jump up and down at this seemed appropriate, but caution prevailed. My prostate cancer doctor was not an ENT specialist and he was not privy to all the medical information pertinent to my case history; though he had done a stint on throat cancer, he was still not a specialist. However, he had given us hope. Hope before Christmas was the best present my family and I were given, which we gladly appreciated. Confusion was a state of mind that prevailed regarding who was right, who was wrong, but within me, I felt a feeling of hope, and if there was a hint of hope, then there was a possibility that I faced a lesser medical issue. We thanked the doctor, departed and headed for home, dwelling on this information. Grace had a reserved smile on her face, but nonetheless a smile; as for me, I kept mine hidden, as I tended to do.

A telephone call continued the day's eventful nature, offering me an earlier operation appointment on Monday January 5, 2015 instead of the original appointment July 2015. It seemed everything was working in my favour all of a sudden in a strange kind of way. It did place additional pressure on us over Christmas, but we had been there before. It was very important that I stayed as fit as possible and increased my lung capacity by exercising more. This would assist me during my operation, as there were high risks associated with this operation. It was a rather subdued Christmas and New Year's celebration for my family, since everyone was worried, especially now that the operation was to take place sooner rather than later. Christmas passed very quickly, as did the New Year's celebrations; soon, the day of the operation dawned. With prayers said and much air in my lungs, I arrived at the hospital for my operation. I had had my pre-op assessment three days prior, which came back as good to go, so I supposed I was as ready as I could be.

The concern was that, with my physical size and weight, anything untoward could happen in this operation. However, I was in the hands of God and in His hands my life was placed, because I had faith and trust in Him (I knew everything would turn out okay).

I reported to the hospital Monday January 5, at 07:00 hours, and my operation commenced a few hours later. I recall returning to this world at 16:10 hours in some discomfort and pain as they called my name again and again. Their hazy faces in front of my eyes were nothing more than that as they requested things of me and I opted not to comply. After a few minutes, I felt that I could comply and gradually did so. What remained firmly etched in my mind was the loss of time; I had no recollection of anything whatsoever in my suspended state between 12:50 hours and 16:10 hours, not even a dream, but zilch, nothing, nothing at all. The oxygen mask placed over my mouth and instructions to inhale was all I recalled before wham, out stone cold.

16:10 hours was the time I returned to the world of reality. Grogginess, pain, soreness and mild disorientation were some of the feelings I experienced as I tried to focus on where and who I was as I lay in a recovery room bed. Around me were medical staff and other patients, as well as a hive of activity, most of which I recall, surprisingly enough. As the nurses gave me varying instructions, I gave nods rather than verbal responses, which made sense as compared to dealing with the pain that would pluck away at my throat area if I talked.

For the next two hours, I remained in the recovery room, waiting to recover sufficiently to be transferred back to the ward. In fact, I was the last patient to leave the recovery bay room due to an ECG trace error showing up and a slight concern from the anaesthetist. Once clear, I was wheeled back to my ward and in no time, my eldest daughter and my partner surrounded me. This placed a painful semi-smile on my face, but inside, I was overjoyed at seeing them. Most importantly, I survived the operation, a reality about which doubt had been raised due to my weight and oxygen capacity. They both remained with me for about one hour before departing the ward, as I needed sleep and rest after such an exhausting day.

As I lay there, in my mind, I thanked God for watching over me and guiding the surgeons' hands, as well as all medical staff involved. I sunk into a deep sleep for a few hours before the nurses disturbed my temporary moment of rest to take my vitals. So it went on for the ensuing ten hours of 'disturbed sleep.'

Tuesday morning arrived quickly and I found myself walking around by its early hours. I was still in some discomfort and unsteady on my feet, but able to shuffle around to keep my legs from going to sleep and DVT at bay.

At approximately 08:00 hours, like military clockwork precision, the consultant arrived on the ward to carry out his rounds. It just so happened that I was walking by the nurses' station upon his arrival, and he decided to stop me and examine the area upon which he had operated. He commented that he was happy and, subject to blood test results, I could go home later. A smile came to my face, but nothing like the smile that came when he, having physically examined the partial thyroid removed, revealed that, in his opinion, he felt that it was not cancerous, but the histology would confirm that over the next few days. I was elated beyond a doubt; the thunderstorm that was looming over me had now become a rainbow as, at long last, some luck had come my way. Deep down, I knew I would be fine; I knew it. I immediately started texting family and friends about the news, perhaps somewhat prematurely, but I simply had to share the good news. They deserved it because, if you feed the happiness, then the sadness will starve.

Chapter 10 - The LAST Diary Entry 2015

February 10, 2015

This will be the last of my diary recollections for this book. I am due at the Mount Vernon Cancer Treatment Centre at 11:30 hours for my monthly consultation review. As usual, I feel apprehensive, even after almost three years of attendance. I awoke at 06:50 hours mainly because my partner departs for work, waking me up for our ritual morning kiss and a few words. At around 09:00 hours, my first set of tablets was taken: four x abiraterone plus one x Prednisolone on an empty stomach.

An hour later, the second set of tablets was taken with my breakfast. This has been the ritual, as you are aware, for the past three years. Nearing 11:30 hours, I arrived at the hospital and parked my car in the hospital car park. As I looked in my bag for my discounted coin that allowed me to park at a reduced rate, I could not help but wonder how hospital administrations could charge cancer patients for parking, regardless of the subsidy. The financially impaired among us need every penny, let alone every pound. It all just adds to the stress. You administrators say you understand. I say, "Do you really?" Consider this: a patient that attends a hospital twice a month (sometimes more if scans and other medical procedures are required) for three years must pay a pretty sum. This is a sum that could be used for more vital items. It's just my opinion, though; dwell on that, you thinkers and planners.

Anyway, I checked in with reception and waited in the waiting room area of the chemotherapy suite. As I sat there, I noted other people around me, similarly waiting for their appointments. I began to wonder to myself, "What sorts of cancer do they have? What stage is their cancer at?" It also made me wonder about the huge amount of worrying that went on in this world-famous cancer treatment centre, the accumulated fear, the loss and distress.

You can only guess about it, looking around the waiting rooms. You see patients and relatives, some appearing weak, some stressed, but the seasoned ones (that's me included) chat merrily, throwing in a smile every now and then over their coffee, ginger beer or hot chocolate.

As I sat there, varying conversations were within my earshot. Some talked about the pain medications they were on and the side effects they were causing. Some talked about family and how someone was pissing them off. Some talked about hospital procedures with which they were not happy. Some just sat in silence, like I did, and observed. On this occasion, I attended my appointment by myself because it was becoming too time consuming for Grace and the family to attend with me, only to really hear the regular verdict that all was well with me. As I sat there, one gentleman came out of a consultation room, shuffling around and looking dazed. It was though the medication he was on was affecting his walking ability, an effect I had undergone and knew only too well. Another gentleman looked agitated as he sat with his jaw rested on his hands, as if he was pensively pondering pensively something or another.

I wanted to go over and ask him if all was well and if I could do anything for him. However, I decided against it. I had done the same on previous occasions, only for patients to want to be left alone, so I refrained. My appointed time came and I was summoned into the nurse's consultation room. As usual, pleasantries were exchanged and the usual questions asked of me. These included the common "How have you been since we last met? Any planned or unplanned hospital visits?" lines, among others.

She proceeded to inform me of my latest PSA results. "Mr. Samuels, once again, your reading is less than 0.1ng/ml and all your other bloods taken are good. You're doing well." So there, I rest my anxiety and anticipation for yet another month. Next, my blood pressure was taken, but it seemed not to want to register a level reading; it took four attempts before the nurse was happy. I knew the cause was my stress over travelling to the hospital, as well as my bout of heavy sweating I had just undergone while in her office. She shunted off to see the consultant and I was made to wait in the waiting room again.

There, I was greeted by a set of new faces that had just arrived for their appointments. Though they might not have been new to the waiting room area, they were new to me. One gentleman paused his reading as I entered and looked up at me. I nodded and gave a smile, and, lo and behold, I got a smile in return. Well, there's another waiting room buddy for me, I suppose. Waiting for their appointments it is, as if there is a common facial expression bordering on a mask that people exhibit. As thumbs twiddled and rolled, hands twitched and legs tapped out of rhythm, all showing signs of anxiety and worry.

Around me were posters regarding cancer, free prescriptions for cancer patients and a multitude of other information. There was nothing to take one's mind away or off of thinking about cancer. Again, I wondered if the powers that be understood the psychosocial impact this has. My personal boundaries between physical and mental health, however, are paper-thin. My need for time off has been due not only to the physical effects of cancer treatments, but also to the huge psychological and psychosocial emotional adjustments I have had to make, especially where my consultancy business was concerned.

Tonight I chatted within an online group on Prostate Cancer UK. Whilst chatting with one guy, we realised that we both had gone through the same treatment process and how it had affected us mentally and emotionally. In his own word he said "I was on that trial and it did the same to me, after six months I got pulled off it, before I harmed myself badly. Also being single didn't help as I found myself in the darkness, which wasn't good, but Macmillan buddies were very good to talk too. I am now on antidepressants. Life settled down still get bad days but better now. What's funny all I can remember is I had very dark periods, but can't remember what happened. **I recall**

interjecting and saying, really....oh I remembered mine because I kept a diary and when it went wrong I wrote it down....So its in ink for me....He replied with I just couldn't write it down I lost the will power to do anything. Even got sent to see a group called MIND and psychologist along with hypnosis. I am feeling better in myself now and still coping with working full-time.

I could only read in astonishment at his statement because, it was as if I was looking in the mirror, at what I had gone through but without the medication, group therapy and Psychologist.

The following morning I awoke feeling very strange and actually felt unwell.

I found I could not stop thinking about last nights conversation, and asked myself the question, had it affected me that much? Then the penny dropped, had my emotional memory being jogged by the exchange with my online buddy, and was my body coming out in sympathy, it seemed so. As I laid in bed carrying out mental reframe time, I concluded that I needed to explore later emotional triggers that could have physical manifestations. If not identified they could catch me off guard and at the very least, unknowingly affect my energy and physical levels.

It may be stormy inside my head here at the moment, but it can't rain forever. I just need to remember that courage does not always roar. Sometimes, courage is a quiet voice at the end of the day saying, "Just try again tomorrow, Alfred, just try again."

Chapter 11 – My Partner & Family

It should be quite clear by now that I have gone through an avalanche of feelings during my illness and, without the love of my family, I probably would not have survived. Grace, you and you alone cared for me unstintingly and made me feel alive; you are so infinitely dear to me, dearer than I can say – I could spend days upon days calling you endearing names and paying you homage and compliments without ever being satisfied. If ever two were one, then surely we were; I love you and you love me, as our two souls stand erect and strong in the face of adversity. You are that extraordinary woman. Even during the darkest days, you and certain members of the family showed me that there were rays of sunshine just waiting to burst through.

On Good Friday of 2014, Grace became ill and I had to rush her to the hospital. She was suffering from stomach pains that literally doubled her over. As we sat in the hospital waiting room, reminders of my time in this less than slumberous place flashed through my mind. She clutched my hand as we sat and I felt every painful jerk that shuddered through her body. Her eyes were red with tears of pain and agony from what she was going through at that moment in time. For the first time medically in our relationship, it was not about me, as the worried expression on her face showed. I knew it was serious and I had not planned or foreseen this eventuality. Grace, become ill? Never, ever, not my 'iron lady,' but she was. In less than three hours from our arrival at A&E and examination, she was admitted for serious internal issues.

Now it was my turn to stand up tall and strong in the face of her adversity. Surgery was mentioned and the stark reality of the situation became clearer: it was my turn to care for her and, without much ado, I did. Calls were immediately made to her son Joshua and sisters Bev and Carol, apprising them of the situation. Painkillers, antibiotics, anti-inflammatory tablets and an IV drip were all given to her as hospital staff tried to ascertain what was wrong. I was worried; in fact I was more than worried, I was frightened. What if I lost my Grace, my right arm? I realised I was falling into a pessimistic state of mind in front of her. My mood and demeanour changed, and my alpha male dominance engaged. I now had to be the strong one to care for her and her son.

My condition became a secondary concern and was pushed to the back of my mind. As we conversed, it was clear she was more concerned about the two men in her life. I reassured her that we would manage and that I would take care of her son, no matter what happened. She smiled at my words, as it was clear they went a long way toward alleviating her main worry. However, within me, tears were flooding my mind at the thought of her demise. Her admission was a real turning point in our relationship and I was strong enough to endure what was ahead. She remained in hospital for seven days and each day, twice a day I visited her without fail, ensuring all her needs were met. She looked awful, frail, weak and still wincing in pain throughout most of my visits. Her family rallied around her; her son, sisters and elderly mother were all there. This alleviated some pressure on me, but my emotions were all over the place nonetheless.

If she had died, I would have been devastated; I know in my heart of hearts that I would not have recovered. I had to keep these negative thoughts out of my mind and show her the uplifting face of healing. During her stay one evening, at around 23.00 hours I received a surprise call from her at home. I had only left her two hours earlier. Her weak, yet audible voice carried from the speaker and what she said next caused the veins in my neck to stand out in rage. She barely had time to put the phone down before I was at the hospital and in no time on the ward. It turned out that, earlier in the day, a cannula had been taken out of her arm and no one had returned to resite it, which meant she was not receiving the IV antibiotics into her blood stream.

Grace is a fully trained and qualified nurse and fully conversant with medical procedures.

I located the ward sister and informed her of the telephone call I received and its nature. The sister assured me that she would personally deal with the matter. Given the situation, she really had no option; a six-foot unsmiling alpha male with a good command of English had diplomatically informed her that shit was going to hit the fan if something was not corrected. I was fully prepared to take it to the next level if cooperation was not forthcoming. They were hurting my loved one and I was not going to sit there and knowingly allow this. They had woken a sleeping lion but thankfully it did not come to that and matters were resolved. The following day, a complaint was filed with the doctor and there, the matter ended.

You hear of these weird stories within the NHS, but never expect them to befall you, do you? Come on, it's 23.00 hours at night and I have to attend a female ward? As I have said before in this book, what the fuck, NHS, get a grip. People are dying because of incompetent staff on our wards. Each day I visited her, I felt her pain and it entwined with my own, causing my stress levels to increase. I found that I had started to fall into a state of disrepair.

Nevertheless, I had made a promise to her that I would look after everything, so I quickly snapped out of that state. Her consultant at the hospital was thorough, considerate, gentle and empathetic to her condition, which was very much female-orientated. He reassured us that all would be well and after seven days, she was discharged and returned home. It did not stop there for me because now was a time for recuperation before she would be able to return to anywhere near her former self. My voice could be heard on many occasions, ordering my iron lady to rest. Josh played his part when he could. Because he was at university, he was not always around, but between us, we managed her recuperation well.

A reflective moment came after she returned home, when I talked with the man above and asked Him to take me instead of her. I would have gladly exchanged my life for hers if this was the only course open to us, but we did not have to travel that avenue. I thanked Him for sparing her and nursing her back to full health, though I wondered what His plan was for me after this traumatic episode that befell us.

Yes, many a time I have wondered how our relationship would have been if the circumstances were different. But it will relieve you to know nothing would be any different in my eyes. You are like my child, my little wife, my angel and my best friend, all rolled into one. I promise you that God sparing that my name will be due to you From day one I wanted to prepare you for the inevitable, not realising that I would come out the other side still whole, though scathed and mentally scared.

I could never forget how much you have done for me, I could never forget how much you unconditionally loved me, and I could not ever forget you. My children, and that includes you, Joshua, have all made me feel so proud as you played your parts equally. I, as a father, am so proud of you all, in all that you have achieved so far and the possibilities to be. Your messages of support, your voices over the telephone, our quality moments spent, and boisterous restaurant nights, our shopping trips, which emptied my wallet, and your personal visits were all integral to my will and desire to live and to never, ever give up.

I know one day I will have to leave you all, but always know this: there is a spiritual afterlife and I will always be there among you all. My family, Kelly, my younger brother , you saw it before anyone else when you lifted me into your car, when I could move no more. You watched over me when the pain was unbearable, but you stayed strong; though you cried on the inside, you kept your emotions intact.

When times were hard, you were my guardian angel; mum and dad would have been proud of you. Doreen, my baby sister, mum lead you to God before she left us and you have never veered from that path. How little did I know one day I would need to call on you, and you never let me down when I came a-calling.

To the cancer medical staff, especially at Mount Vernon Hospital, who administered my most recent care and all the Macmillan nurses, wherever you are, a tremendous and hearty thank you to you all. I know that things within the NHS are not perfect and, at times, unbearable, but you all make it work nonetheless. My local hospital oncology department you started caring for me, though we parted under questionable circumstances. Prior to my complaint, I again applaud you for that time of care.

Sadness in general is a difficult feeling to curb, but the traumatic diagnosis of cancer is a far deeper feeling to undertake. The melancholy caused by this deep feeling clearly interfered with my day-to-day life and, at times, left me feeling unmotivated and even worthless. There were periods when my mental stability became questionable, so much so that I had confided with Grace.

I now understand how people can get to the depths of despair and take their lives, having contemplated taking my own. About a year into my illness, I was invited out to an event at a prestigious hotel in central London. The event was held on the twentieth floor and I attended with Grace. It was nice to be actually out among people, something I had not managed to do for many, many months. I'm not really a socialite and actually prefer my own and my partner's company. Nonetheless, we attended, mingled and tried to show our cheerful sides.

At some stage during the evening, we found ourselves on the balcony of this hotel penthouse suite, looking out into the skyline of central London and all that it has to offer. As I stood there with Grace, I bowed my head quietly, not saying much between us, but with much going on in my head. Here I was, walking the road others had paved, trying to say to myself and to others I was fine and really knowing I was not. Hoping that the tears of others would stop, I manifested a plan of unimaginable proportions. At that moment with my head bowed, I wished, I prayed I was someone else without cancer, but I was not. I was me, who had cancer.

I looked up and my eyes gazed on Grace in her infinite beauty as she stood there. She looked so beautiful as she smiled at me in her inquisitive way; she was questioning "is everything fine?" Tears came to my eyes as they veered off to her left, towards the edge of the balcony into the dark depths of suicide. Many other thoughts circled my mind; I did not want to continue living in constant pain, filling my body every day with medications, lethargy, weight gain due to steroid tablets, hair loss. That's what chemotherapy tablets had done to me; I never in a million years dreamed that my life could end up this way. It was certainly no way to live or continue to live.

But before me was a way out. I said to myself, "It's easy, just take two or three steps, hurl your body over and the pain will stop forever." Let me tell you, even as I write these words, my legs are trembling, as I recalled that moment of crazy insanity. I froze in that spot when the thought came to my mind that night; my heart immediately started to pump faster and harder and I could not talk. It seemed like an eternity had passed before I heard my angel's words: "Al, are you okay?" I replied, "No, I am not, let's get off this balcony."

With Grace behind me, I literally clung to the building's window ledge and pigeon-stepped back into the safety of the penthouse suite.

Grace's face looked perplexed as my face showed much was wrong. I was sweating profusely and my heart was pumping even harder and faster, like an athlete after a sprint event. To still remain here standing and able to share this event with you while so many others have fallen is in itself a miracle. Disbelief, fear, despair and anxiety came in quick succession, jumbled up, back and forward, again and again in my head as I replayed what had just unfolded.

For me, mentally, this was the moment when the cancer gained control and was not loosening its hold on me. This evil, cruel disease that I had vowed to fight was at this moment in time ahead and winning. It had sapped me of all my energy and diminished my strength, but in front of me was my tower of strength, my Grace, and I had to tell her what had transpired. I held her hand as I told myself I needed to confide in her, and we moved away to a quieter location within the suite.

Grace listened with empathy at first, then, as it became clearer what my intention was, her face became mortified. She became greatly concerned at what she was hearing.

I cannot reiterate enough that cancer is very much a mental thing; survivability requires a cast iron will and determination if one is to stand any reasonable chance of getting through.

Obviously, medication also plays a great part in the healing process. However, if your mental attitude is one of giving up before the first mouthful of pills is swallowed, you are beaten in the race of life. Our duly elected governments have a duty of care. Cures for many illnesses have been found over the past years and, one day, I am sure that a cure for cancer will be found, but only if significant research funding is made available. Cancer does not discriminate and it can only be to society's advantage to find a cure, because otherwise, it could be you or yours next.

As things currently stand, you have to assume you will get cancer at some stage in your life, hopefully in a curable form. Everyone's cancer journey is different. Anyone with an illness of any kind is just happy that someone cares enough to take time out for them. Family, friends and people genuinely mean well when it comes to offering a cancer sufferer support, telling you "I know how you feel."

The truth is, you never really do. If you have been through a cancer experience, you may have an understanding, but unless you are going through the cancer sufferer's identical experience, you have no idea what they are experiencing. I once read an article that said, "You should not play doctor, as the cancer sufferer has at least one of those." Personally speaking, if I want information, I'll ask for it. I am already inundated with information and advice from medical personnel, so your two pennies' worth about an article from a newspaper, magazine or online publication is not necessary.

You all want to help and that's very admirable, but the stories of your mother/grandmother/sister/aunt/friend who had cancer can, at times, remind me of someone else, for example, my own mother, aunt, uncle and cousins, if you can understand that. Also, telling me a story about your family member or friend who has had cancer is simply irrelevant. It's especially a bad idea if it's a fatal story; it does not help me to process my diagnosis or make decisions about my own cancer treatment.

Please do not take this the wrong way or think I am bashing you when I ask if you really understand what you are saying when you utter statements to me along the lines of "how are you feeling?" Yes, the phrase may show that you care, but so many people have asked me the same question and it gets really old and flaming annoying after a while. Many, many a time, I did not feel so great and being asked that question only reminded me of that.

The words "You're strong and will get through it" suggested to me that I needed to be tough to survive, and that's not necessarily true. I always preferred to hear the words "I'm sorry you're ill and I'm/were thinking of you." Gestures such as taking me to one of my clinical treatment appointments or cooking me a meal speak louder than words.

They say misery loves company; however, misery does not always love the positive spin on tragic life events. Just remember, every cancer patient has a different opinion and experience of what they are going through. You can't feel their pain and no two tales are ever the same, just because a common word is the link.

My weight at diagnosis was 121kg; after three years of treatment, it shot up to 133kg, in part due to the required daily use of steroid tablets. During the late months of 2014, I decided that the pains were virtually non-existent, therefore it was time to concentrate on my fitness level. I needed something that would stretch me, but not overwork me, as this was to be a gradual process of regaining some level of fitness. Subsequently, I was introduced to Northala Hills on the Western Avenue of the A40 Greater London, Middlesex.

Northala Fields is an award-winning country-style park and consists of four artificial hills, you'd be forgiven for wondering if the four hills are actually ancient burial mounds, forts or landing pads for alien spaceships.

Along with Grace, whose fitness level was also lacking, we decided to kill two birds with one stone by climbing these four separate hills. Our view was that climbing these hills between twice and three times each week would rapidly increase our fitness levels. Well, on the first hill that we attempted to climb, I found it extremely hard going, leaving us feeling breathless and winded after the first hill, with no desire, energy or vision to even move downwards back to ground level or on to the next hill.() Surprisingly, Grace had reached the top of the first hill and was spurring me on. With this incentive, I trudged away and made it, but my vision was blurred, my legs were robotic and I was gasping for air upon reaching the peak. After a short rest, we decided to push onto hill two, as it seemed pointless to come all the way only to ascend one hill. From previous military experience, I knew that walking down a hill could also be quite challenging if approached in the wrong way. I could risk joint damage, especially in the ankle and knee areas. I used a short zigzag method (actually kind of like skiing) as I descended; plunging heels-first downward worked great and I reached ground level again.

As we pushed on, I recall Grace being ahead of me, which helped me immensely, as I had someone and something to aim at as we pushed upwards again. 'Left, right, left, right, left, right' were the words etched and flowing freely through my mind as my feet planted themselves into the ground with each stride. Puffing and panting with Grace slightly ahead, we reached the hilltop. By now, my lungs were screaming and my mouth desirous of liquid.

I recall Grace telling me to slow my breathing down; "Slow it down," she repeated, which I complied with and found that my screaming for air soon ceased. Soon afterward, I started to recover more quickly. I knew the process of slow breathing to recoup, but damned if I remembered at the time to do it.

Grace was actually fitter and better than me at this, but then again, no surprise there, considering the situation. After a little rest, we descended hill two, but my mind had already been defeated in any attempt to climb hill three, let alone hill four.

So there we stopped with two hills climbed, proud of ourselves nonetheless. The only question now was whether we could keep this routine up. When looking at these hills from afar, one is mentally reluctant to even consider it, let alone do it. We both agreed that there was easiness in our minds and bodies similar to that of a visit to a spa centre's sauna steam room.

Well, I decided that there was no way that these hills would beat me just like the cancer. As such, over the next month, more frequently than Grace, I trudged up and down those hills until I was comfortably climbing ascending and descending all four. My mindset was that, if I could conquer these by myself, I could conquer anything. As my confidence increased and my fitness grew, I added a Bergen to my back with a light weight inserted, and was able to carry myself up and over all four hills.

I had arrived; I had no reservations or hesitations about the weak feelings about which I had complained so often in my diary over the past few years. I had even seen the physical shape of my thighs coming back; as the flabbiness changed into muscle, I truly was 'coming out the other side.' Grace complemented me by saying she was so proud of me, as it was by no means an easy task. Nevertheless, I had managed to do it, just like how I tackled the cancer. Once I set my mind and goal on something, I generally go onto to achieve it.

Was I going to let a few little old hills stand in my way after all the suffering I had undergone with cancer? No way, no way, mind over matter prevailed. In addition, the strength others around me gained from this was evident. Grace was there on many occasions and her physical health started to improve, as did the strength in her legs. It got to the point that, even with the weighted rucksack on my back, I was bounding up and down these hills ahead of Grace. I found that I was no longer feeling as tired as I had felt over many months. That's not to say the fatigue had disappeared fully, but now I had the energy to fight the exhaustion.

A few months prior, I would never have contemplated such a feat. I recall mentioning this to one of my doctors, who was thrilled about my hill walking, commenting, "You're a determined kind of person anyway, so I expected nothing less." I found much freedom once I had reached the top of these hills and looked out yonder and above.

Maybe it was the feeling of being nearer and closer to God. Nothing inhibited me; though I was clothed, I felt truly naked and free of all stresses, pains and ailments in my mind. It may have been for a moment, but you know something? Even a moment of total freedom is worth more than gold.

Well, it's September 2014 and, at long last, we have booked our holiday, a cruise. It will be my first cruise, but Grace's sixth, nonetheless a well-deserved holiday for both of us. We booked a 10-day cruise out of Miami, Florida, U.S., covering the Eastern Caribbean islands of St. Thomas, St. Martin and Nassau in the Bahamas. Grace is overly excited about it and, in many ways, so am I. Both our bodies yearn for that tropical sun. Though my sweating will be an issue, I'm not going to let it spoil our first real overseas holiday together.

Having looked through the brochures, the pictures looked great, as did the Norwegian cruise liner vessel "The Getaway." The vessel featured advantageous components such as a balcony cabin for us to share. I intended to rest, as did my partner. No work, no computers, no phones. I have also decided to just eat seafood and salads for the 10-day voyage, the former being one of my favourites. I have heard differing opinions with regard to cruises, and now, I will experience one for myself. I hoped and prayed that my cancer would not limit or inhibit me in any way from enjoying the cruise. Ideally, this would serve as a break from the confinement of my home and four walls, which at times felt like an incarceration sentence. I know it's my home, but it reminded me so much of my illness at times that I felt like I needed to run away.

The build up to this holiday was fraught with anticipation and worry for us both, especially as the travel insurance did not allow for cancer health issues. Cruises that set sail prior to or during the holiday are not cheap, I can tell you. Well, the months became weeks and the weeks became days until our departure date from the UK. For me, two things marred our vacation as they did Grace. Firstly, our flight on an Airbus A300 was the coldest flight that I personally have ever taken in my entire life. The air conditioning system was absolutely freezing, so much so that virtually all passengers on board wore jackets, hooded tops, and cardigans, as well as utilising on board blankets. When I questioned a cabin crewmember, he told me "That's just how it is on these flights."

I was amazed, dumbstruck to be precise, that cancer patients and cold weather do not go well together (not to say that the airline knew my circumstances). Nine hours and thirty-five minutes did not put me in the right state of mind for my holiday break (I sent a letter of complaint). Secondly, upon our arrival at the hotel, our reservation was not registered. To say I was hopping mad would be an understatement, but getting myself into an irate mood would not do me any good, so I left it to Grace to sort out. After a forty-five minute wait and frantic calls from the Virgin travel representative to the hotel, matters were resolved and our holiday commenced.

For me personally, our holiday was very much about smiles, holding hands, reigniting our love for each other and simply resting our weary minds and bodies. The wellness in our faces reflected our jubilation at taking a chance with this holiday. After much walking during our holiday and the exhausting heat, my feet gave way the day before we docked back in Miami, which was a shame. Both my feet swelled up and became very painful to walk on, and I felt a constant smarting for most of the night into the early morning. I recall talking to my oncologist upon my return and telling him about my feet, to which they answered they were not surprised, especially after the heat we had been in. For me, that was the only pain I felt for the total duration of our holiday, for which I was eternally thankful.

Pain-free moments in my life were rarities scarcely felt these last three years. I'm still very sensitive to issues of cancer on a whole; watching and listening to TV programmes or commercials about said subject puts me in a sullen mood for those moments in time. During the month of October 2014, I visited my doctor, whom I had requested refer me to the Macmillan nurses. I felt that I needed to make use of their invaluable service instead of constantly bombarding my partner with certain pertinent questions. It took almost eight weeks for this to happen, eight weeks, I ask you, and then the referral was to a hospice. To say I was disappointed would be an understatement; the mere mention or thought of the word 'hospice' suggested a final moment and I certainly was not there. I recall telling Grace and my oncologist, who made a funny remark: "You feel like you just want to deck him, don't you?" This was a cockney term that meant 'to strike someone on the chin and see them collapse onto the floor.'

My oncologist was good at putting a smile on my face at times, but still, I felt troubled by any inference to the word 'cancer' or associated ones; maybe I will never get over this.

There is not a morning that I have woken that I have not sat on the edge of my bed, reflecting on my prostate cancer disease. For twenty to thirty minutes, I would just sit and float into my own world, trawling through the aftermath I faced after the initial diagnosis, not to mention the treatment and after effects to date.

The notion that this was the end of my life as I knew it has obviously changed from January 2012 to January 2015; the treatment was administered and my body and mind coped with itI suppose the main change has been how psychologically resilient I have become in coping with this disease. My resilient attitude has not meant that I have been forced into thinking positively all of the time. Far from that, the added stress of debt, daily business matters and family issues caused deep anxiety and depressive moments. My mood swings of sadness, loneliness and anger were part of my daily chores, but I never really felt that there was anything wrong about going through these emotions.

There were occasional happy moments and days that I felt great, and I felt totally positive towards life. These were the days that I found myself bargaining for survival with a higher being; these were my happy and enlightening days. As time progressed, I found that I had to come up with a coping strategy that covered the medical, comfort and psychosocial areas of support. Throughout my cancer treatment, I noticed that differing people regularly surrounded me, be they professional, such as doctors, research nurses, surgeons and clergy, or family and friends. All of these interactions involved a whirlwind of emotions and racing thoughts taking me over at any one time.

I found that, for me to cope that, I had to create a two-sphere group. The first treatment I received had a devastating effect on my thought process and feelings in terms of my ability to withstand the entire course of treatment ahead of me. On reflection, I wondered how I did it. The first series of clinical trials, the first relapse and all of the on-going changes in my personal life I endured made me feel like I was chasing a moving target.

What is clear to me now is that the cancer process is actually a series of challenges and obstacles that had to be overcome for me to move on to the next phase or challenge. Sometimes, these adjustments became so overwhelming that it was difficult to see the light at the end of the tunnel. While the initial diagnosis raised the worst fear in my mind, with the advent of the prostate treatment abiraterone, it was becoming clear that a diagnosis of cancer was not always fatal.

Being told you have cancer is something no one wants to hear. When the news is given, you instantly think that you're on a clock. My cancer journey started in a less-than-appropriate manner and in a less-than-appropriate setting.
My mother, aunt, uncle and cousin's demise had unknowingly impacted me greatly and had to be dealt with separately, as they occurred at different stages in my life.

Having entered the realm of depression and contemplated suicide without seeking help, I had left the door of uncertainty wide open, allowing in further fears, issues and experiences related to adjusting to my cancer process vulnerability. There were times I wondered if normalcy would come back in full or in part.

I believe I had an extremely high tolerance level for the physical symptoms associated with treatments, such as pain, nausea and fatigue. They felt so devastating at times, tending to linger on and on. Even today, fatigue hinders the greatest part of my recovery process. Hence, when the window of opportunity came and I felt well enough to re-engage in normal life activities, I jumped at the chance to bring a sense of normalcy back in my life, even if only for a short while. All in all, I found I had more strength than I thought I had, but maybe we all have that strength when faced with adversities. We just need to dig deep to bring it to the surface.

I have further realised as time progressed that the place you go to obtain medical treatment can also bring about a condition I refer to as a state of anxiousness when attending and receiving treatment. I was always anxious a few days before or when sitting in front of my oncologist or research nurse, waiting for blood test results in relation to my PSA. These would indicate how well I was doing or not doing.

One of the worst side effect changes for me was when I realised I was not functioning mentally correctly and, at times, talked total gibberish, looking confused and feeling unclear as to where I actually was. Sometimes, I simply just walked around and around in circles. It was only when I visited my GP and consultant that it became clear the combined strength of the medications were causing these side effects within me. This further distress on the whole just further frustrated and challenged me. My thought process during my illness lead me to the understanding – do not fear death! Why? Because it's inevitable; we are all born to die. Death is a natural part of life's progression; however, anxiety about this is a built-in survival instinct that surfaces when certain triggers are activated.

Cancer backed me into a corner and tried to stop me from seeing a way out. I recall talking with my children while they were growing up, telling them not to back away from anything that seemed tough. Overcoming adversities would allow them to grow and evolve as individuals.

The next challenge they came across would make them stronger. "Don't give up" is what I would always say and here I was now, looking back at my words.

There were times I felt like giving up, but then, within me, that meant

I did not have any respect for myself. It was as if I were saying that I was not good enough. With that in mind, I knew that the feeling could live with me and possibly come into play with any future decisions I made down the line.

Chapter 12 Crossroads

After a few weeks of provoking thoughts, I decided that the time had come to take myself off the stampede trials drug programme. I had now been on the trials programme for three painstaking years, attending it once, sometimes twice a month during this period. I was undergoing severe financial hardship during this time and felt that, should this continue, my mental stability would come into question. I had previously raised the question of altering my monthly attendance to between six to eight weeks, but the trial committee procedure did not allow for this, as there were stringent guidelines. After allowing a few months to pass and giving the matter much thought, I decided now was the time to state my case and put my foot down, as I could take myself off this trial programme at any time.

I discussed the matter with family and found a split among them that caused me to rethink my decision. I always consulted them in do-or-die decision-making processes, though ultimately, it was my decision in the end. My inability to work or travel without undue concern for appointments was now paramount in my mind.

After further thought, I made a firm decision to come off the trial and constructed an email to the oncology department of Mount Vernon Hospital. I advised them, should they fail to reconsider my situation, then I would be left with no alternative but to withdraw from the programme. My email went as follows:

"11th February 2015

Att: - Mount Vernon Hospital

Ref: - Stampede Drugs Trials Patient NHS No. xxxxxxxxxxxxxxxxxxxx

I trust that my email finds you well today. Allow me to get straight to the point. As you know, I attended the clinic yesterday for my routine consultation and during my visit, I revisited the issue of my monthly attendance at the "Stampede Drugs Trials Programme," in which I have been a participant for the past three years, as you know.

I raised the question of whether I could vary my required monthly attendance to between six to eight weeks, a time scale that would allow me to travel internationally and easily fulfil any of my work contracts. You advised me that the trial committee procedure rules do not allow for this to happen due to the stringent guidelines in keeping a check on certain medical procedures as laid down. The past 18 months have seen a steady set of results showing that the disease is under control, returning not only PSA values of less than 0.1 each month, but also no issues with any other blood function test carried out. With this in mind, I am now attempting to revive my consultancy business, which has been caused serious financial hardship over the past few years.

The question now arises as to what the procedure would be for me to "sign off the Stampede Drugs Trials programme" and in doing so, what medical implications this would entail. A further question would be whether I could sign off for a limited period of time, say four to six months, and then sign back on. I would appreciate a reply with a possible workable solution, as I am being left with no option but to sign off the programme. There does not seem to be any leeway afforded to me in accommodating the mental anguish facing me due to finances. I look forward to your imminent reply."

The reply to my email came in the form of a telephone conversation; at my next consultation appointment, the matter would be discussed in full. I felt that this was reasonable, especially because, as the month was currently February, we could talk the matter over in March, making my involvement in the trials programme exactly three years. For the first time in our relationship, Grace and I were not unified in a decision, nor was my son James, which made matters worrying. The majority of my children agreed with me and understood I was doing what I had to do. Grace and James, however, differed and felt I was being selfish. Well, I can tell you now my home did not feel like a home for many a week, and the extent to which our relationships would be tested remained to be seen. Let me be totally open and frank about what I was about to do.

By withdrawing from the stampede trails, I was putting my life at risk. No longer would I receive the current abiraterone medication that had been instrumental in lowering my PSA to a virtually undetectable level. As you could see from my email to the oncology department, I was asking for a suitable alternative in lieu of the abiraterone tablets that would grant me more flexibility in appointment attendance. It was my life; I was going through the mental anguish of a man unable to feed his family and my partner as the main breadwinner. It was my whole manliness being questioned far beyond the cessation of sexual function. How could I make her understand all of this? This was the question constantly on my mind; no matter how I tried, my option was not acceptable.

I decided to remain firm and solid in my decision since I knew what was best for my family and me. March came very quickly, as did my appointment, and for the first time in a long while, Grace did not attend my next consultation appointment with me. The feeling of being let down existed, but I respected her decision, once again feeling alone in my journey. Everything from a family perspective had gone so well up until this moment, and a defining moment it was going to be. I attended my appointment and was seen by a registrar who went into my e-mail's subject matter in-depth. He explained that should I decide to withdraw, I would no longer receive the abiraterone tablets and over a short period of time, my PSA would ultimately rise.

The rise would eventually lead to bodily function failure and ultimately death. My simple reply was that I have been there before, so death does not worry me. This took the doctor by surprise, but an acknowledging nod of his head indicated that he was in agreement with me. As I sat there alone, I pointed out to the doctor that my decision had led to an uncomfortable situation at home, hence the reason for Grace not being in attendance.

At this moment in time, it was clear that a stalemate existed. The doctor looked at me and then said, "Let's find a solution." I smiled and in my mind, I thought everyone was on the same page again.

It was suggested to me that an application into the NHS mainstream programme should be completed, so I could be accepted onto their programme. However, I was forewarned there was no guarantee of my acceptance. The paperwork was commenced, but this would take another month before I was informed of a decision, to which I agreed. The atmosphere at home seemed to rescind somewhat after I explained to Grace that a plan of action that coincided with her thoughts and feelings was underway, and although there was no guarantee, it allowed for a sense of normality to return, if even only for a short while. The next few weeks were unsettled in my mind and all I could do was to pray.

A week prior to my next appointment, I received a telephone call from the hospital doctor informing me that my application had been successful, and that I would now receive my abiraterone tablets via the NHS. This would mean that my appointments would now no longer be monthly but bi-monthly. An array of elated, happy and overjoyed feelings came over me, but the best feeling was the return of unity within my family.

However, the situation at hand revealed a clear kink. While I am of a sound enough mind and body to make decisions at this time in my life, there could come a time later down the line where I would not be in a position to do so. This, then, could result in my family making potential decisions for me, and already we had been in a situation where not everyone was in agreement, so then what? Clearly everyone was being honest about their feelings; it was natural for them to feel their own anger and frustration, and sometimes express it too, as was evident. Understanding what I wanted and what was best for me was the bone of contention, and this could only be sorted out if I called a family meeting to sort this out in advance or as best as I could. This, I placed on my to-do list before matters could change.

I recall during my mother's years of treatment in the 1980s that patients were often discouraged from taking an active part in their own care. Times had changed and my family needed to understand that I was now actively involved in my own care. Admittedly, at the initial beginning, I distanced myself from this process, but that was at the beginning when I was not thinking rationally.

On April 7, Grace and I attended my clinic appointment, and the process for changing over to the NHS version of abiraterone tablets was completed. The hardship for me was the feeling of losing family; what I mean is that the doctors and nurses I was assigned on the Stampede Trials were to part ways with me. Now, I would see a different nurse than I was previously assigned every eight weeks. Unless my PSA was raised or there were indications of issues in other blood test results, then I would not see a doctor, and would just be issued the next set of tablets.

We agreed that we would at least say our goodbyes to the trials research nurse and formally pass on our heartfelt appreciation for all that she had done. Though we would occasionally see her, she would no longer be my point of contact nor would she carry out the various medical tests on clinic visits. This was unforeseen and a further price to pay, though it was not to my detriment. For me personally, the majority of my one-on-one dialogues were with my trials nurse, whom I felt played a major role in my cancer care during most of my appointments.

The nursing I was given not only focused on the medical and biological aspects, but also the emotional aspects of my care. Clearly there were the few occasions when I did not mention questions of a sexual nature for fear of my manliness being bought into question. For me, this was clearly where the barriers were placed and, at times, it led to inadequate emotional support for me as a patient. Having been a regular hospital patient, I knew that complaints about poor relationships between health care personnel and patients often existed.

From personal experience, having gone through some of this during the early parts of my treatment care, not all my patient communicative needs were met. Overall, though, during my care at Mount Vernon Hospital, there existed a positive relationship between my health care personnel and myself, and for this I was extremely grateful; it was one less thing over which to stress. Gaps in communication between caregivers and patients can result in decreased quality of care, poor outcomes and dissatisfaction with an already ailing health care system.

When someone listens carefully with empathy and concern, further explaining things clearly and respecting what a patient says, and spends enough time with said patient so they do not feel like a product on a conveyor belt, a harmonious situation prevails for all.

I have often wondered, though, how health care professionals deal with their inner emotional feelings in having to deal with an array of cancer patients for weeks if not years, seeing some survive, but the majority perish.

Outside of work exists their own personal lives, but how do they shut the door on this heartfelt emotional subject and return the following day with all their emotions, skills and psychological aspects of care intact? Professional they may be, but training can only prepare them for so much of what they undergo; after all, they are only human, but I often wonder, though.

During my illness, I experienced limited social interaction and I felt that this impacted me greatly. I should have socially interacted more with those who were in similar situations to mine, but instead, I retreated to deep within my abode. My state of mind was greatly affected day in and day out between 07.00 and 18.45 hours, during which four walls were my company and solitude. I felt alone and isolated during these highly charged emotional moments in my life.

Prior to my diagnosis, life was good, if not great; however, it was a pretty big shock and a lot to absorb when the diagnosis was made. Feeling trapped and accepting that I was never going to be what I was five years ago was even harder for me to comprehend. When I needed someone to talk to and provide me with mental stimulation outside of my immediate family, my options were limited. I have come to realise that interpersonal relationships play an important role in the process of adapting patients to serious illnesses.

My satisfaction with my partner adhering to all my needs was compounded by high empathy and low withdrawal, causing psychological distress. Here I was with a debilitating disability and having to be reliant on others, a gladiator all my life and a pillar of support to all who wanted to lean on me. On a number of occasions, I sought social and interpersonal support from my doctors as well as decisional support, only to be given hospice access before they realised what they had done.

I had placed a great amount of reliance on the patient-physician relationship, assuming that my cancer care delivery would be processed with great significance, but none of this was ever forthcoming.

Clearly, in my mind this was a failure and I believe only of late has this attracted the attention of cancer researchers as they seek to stem negative interaction and to improve patient-physician communication in cancer care. The Stampede Clinical Trials were sensitive to my physical well-being, but not to other important factors, such as my psychosocial state, that played a critical role in determining my functional response to my illness and treatment. I have walked the roads others have paved and tried convincing myself that I was fine, knowing I was not, primarily in the hope that my family's tears would stop. You don't face cancer being brave, crying as your body fights you from inside, knowing there's nowhere left to hide. I have spent timeless moments sitting with my head quietly bowed in my 4x4, wishing and praying that I had someone to talk to one to one. Eventually, this led me to express my feelings through pen and paper; this allowed me to pour out my heart onto page after page, resulting in a feeling of calmness and relief. The evidence is there that the increasing popularity of online video sharing and personal narratives shared through social media are an area of rapid development in communication among cancer survivors. These social media communication efforts clearly aim to use personal stories to reach individuals with serious illnesses. However, there is still no substitute for direct human companionship, as I still try to grasp what is real.

CHAPTER 13 Here & Now

Whatever your reason for reading my book, whether you are a cancer patient, a family member or a friend of a cancer patient or a medical researcher, I hope my book pointed you toward answers to any of the questions you have been asking. If my story was able to convey the emotional upheaval and pain I have felt, then I have achieved my aim. Maybe others will find the inner strength to fight on and beat the disease of cancer. The emotional effects were the trickiest to navigate through. Emotionally, I was spent just from trying to stay alive as I went through a period of second-guessing my survival and deeply questioning why it was me who got cancer.

Eventually, I learned that my battle with cancer was my own battle. My battle was not the same as anyone else's and I learned not to compare myself with others who have fought, who are fighting or will fight cancer.

Shortly after the treatment commenced, however, I soon realised that I was a survivor and was not relying on some magical moment to pull me through. I also came to realise the depth of courage I possessed, which I never knew before. Who knew I had such grit and tenacity! More than a survivor, I was a warrior. From the moment I was diagnosed, I prayed and looked to God. I did not just hold on to God, I clung to Him because of my late mother and the faith she had when she had cancer. Unbeknown to either of us, she had shown and prepared me years beforehand: the biblical verse that comes to mind when I reflect is verse four of Psalm 23 - Yea, though I walk through the valley of the shadow of death, I will fear no evil; for you are with me; your rod and your staff, they comfort me.

Cancer did not just affect what was happening in my body, it affected my esteem, physical appearance and caused me much stress and anxiety. Merely mentioning the word 'cancer' to people resulted in them talking to you in that funeral-esque tone. I could read what people thought just by the look in their eyes. Some of my friendships changed through this period of my illness; some friendships became stronger, but some disappeared without reason or cause.

I never asked for cancer, but I did seek their friendship; 'bitter,' you say, but I was really just saddened by their lack of understanding and empathy to my dilemma. Some of us can count the amount of friends we have on one hand, and it looks like I have lost my entire hand, as well as numerous friendships.

That being said, some family members were not exempt from this; some tried to impose their own self-importance on me without realising how destructive the values of those self-centered actions were. For me, it was definitely a case of staying away from them or, in certain cases, creating clear boundaries with them. In my mind, they had become energy vampires and the stress of that, along with the energy loss, I could not afford.

Those of us who have been on a 'cancer journey' are transformed in the process, as we tend to see life as sweeter and appreciate it more. Not everybody diagnosed with cancer is able to reach a point where he or she is living free of cancer. People who have never faced illness may not realise it, but life is uncertain (we are born to die) for everyone. Each day is a gift. That's true for everyone, but we as cancer survivors are just more aware of it.

Walking the path of cancer alone is totally inadvisable. In life, we all need someone to lean on, especially in times of crisis. Believe me, cancer is not just a crisis, it's a major catastrophe, probably the worst you will ever face in your life. To date, I have had no direct chemotherapy treatment other than the abiraterone tablets, which are a form of chemotherapy, nor have I had any radiotherapy treatment. That is not to say I will not need radiotherapy treatment in the distant future, but for three years, I have progressed through the treatment plan without the need for this usual part of the treatment.

The abiraterone Stampede Drug Cancer Trials programme has worked for me, for which I am eternally grateful. It gave me hope because, without this, I certainly would have died. My family's love and continual words of encouragement were pitted at times against a white towel of submission, which I wanted to throw in. But deep within me, I found the will and determination to live. Recalling my oncologist doctor's words, "You are a very lucky man. A few years ago you would have gone down very quickly, very quickly indeed." If it were not for the abiraterone tablets acting as a counter offensive, this may well have been the case. Now that life has been temporarily given back to me, I am hopeful that this book will help those suffering from cancer, as well as those about to participate in a cancer treatment programme or research the disease. There is light at the end of the tunnel, and it's not the other light to which I refer. It is Earth's lights.

My focus on my family and business is clearer (family first and foremost, then business) and each day, there is a feeling of achievement as I progress back to my almost former self. Of course, I know full well that I can never be the former me again.

I hope that I have the time to teach my family and pass on the life lessons I have learned. The painful scars of this journey remain etched firmly in my mind, but the feelings of unworthiness, no will or determination nor desire to live are distant memories(. Yes, I was in a world of shit, but I'm alive and I'm not afraid, though I never really was. The Almighty walked next to me throughout the experience, even though moments of doubt did surface. Dealing with cancer was and probably will always be work in progress, because you don't get to choose when cancer comes along. There's no choice, none at all. As for now, I am trying to live my life as close as I can to the one I had; I have not let go of any of my dreams, I have just prioritised. I have ultimately learned that it was vitally important that I kept my emotional feelings hidden. I had learned that exposing my innermost feelings was not unlike an army general giving away battle plans; once my feelings were known, my soul could be subjected to all kinds of attacks.

I am so happy I am in one piece, as my thoughts drift on the few good days and then to the many bad days. It would be wrong of me to say that my thoughts do not fall on a recurrence or flare up of the prostate cancer, but optimistic I will stay that this does not happen. I have said many times throughout this book that love played an integral part of my recovery: the love of my family and friends, the love of my partner and most importantly, the love of myself.

If you do not have love of thyself, then you must hate yourself, and if you hate yourself, your whole recovery process is ill-fated, your chances of survival minimalised further. In addition, allowing your mind to set itself on family and friends not behaving appropriately or considerate to your condition can make you become angry, but remember that anger is only one letter short of DANGER. One must move on from the moment rather than allowing it to linger and cause more pain. It will be you that suffers far greater in the end, not the person that has brought you to this state. I was not always so understanding of anger management as I am today, but only by experiencing am I able to pass on a solution. The weight of anger is far heavier than the weight of joy. It's just human nature. When we are in a state of anger or want to act aggressively towards another, it is usually because we are feeling pain that we have not yet dealt with. Dealing with anger once it arises is a matter of acknowledgement and understanding.

A good friend of mine, who was a government advanced driving instructor, once said something to me, and it has held me in good stead ever since:

"Should you be driving and somebody either cuts you up or demonstrates bad driving skills before you, don't get angry, let it go.

It was a passing moment; the moment has passed, so let it go, it's not worth it."

Financially, a cancer diagnosis and treatment can threaten anyone with bankruptcy and financial ruin, no matter what your earning power is. There are many paths you can take, but they all lead back to the same destination: loss of all resources. When you have cancer, you not only lose who you were - your body no longer looks the same - but you can lose your business, and before you know it, it's a slow downward spiral. For me personally, disability payments did not count for much at all, and I found myself making decisions between purchasing food and paying off some of my bills. Cancer was like a constant heavy weight on my back; finding a way to make that weight lighter was the real battle.

On many occasions, my internal emotions have felt like I was faltering, as if I was sliding down a hillside. It was though the earth around me had given way and I was just trying to claw my way through to keep my head above the deadly life-threatening clogging earth. I was totally unprepared to face the financial costs that still had to be paid, even though I was sick. It just never occurred to me that something would happen to me that could prevent me from being able to work.

I cannot finish my book without taking time out again to say more than thank you to my personal angel, Grace Johnson (my partner) who has taken care of me throughout my illness, and to whom I have so often referred throughout this book. I have praised her, I have admired her strength and endurance, and I have truly cared and loved her in return, not only for me, but for us both. She has said on many an occasion that she did not want recognition for this, but I want to give it to her nonetheless as, initially, I felt that maybe she was too emotionally fragile to deal with the cancer issues that we faced. How wrong I was and how sorry I am for doubting.

On many an occasion, she bore the brunt of my anger and frustration, though she was not the cause of this anger. She was the most trusted person to whom my anger could be vented. Of course, she herself as a loved one was angry about my cancer and how it had impacted and affected our life, which was only natural. I forgot that she, too, was angry and frustrated, and was also having a hard time adjusting. These things, I ignored only too often and, for that, I openly and sincerely apologise.

She listened with her heart and kept the lines of communication open between us, especially during moments when I did not want to think about it, let alone talk about it. Her honest and forthright statements allowed us to make serious decisions far more easily than when they were first presented to us, which aided our fears and worries. Being honest about these feelings allowed us and the family to work through difficult times together, namely because we were unified.

Let me tell you now a diagnosis of cancer changes a family forever. Having cared for my mother along with my other siblings at a younger age, I know what was to be expected, especially if you were very close to that person and the eldest at home. With the tables turned now, cancer caused role changes in our family, and my partner became the head of the household and the main breadwinner. These new responsibilities may have overwhelmed many, but not my partner; she stood solid as a rock throughout. I had heard of many instances where siblings were unable to resolve differences or ill-feelings during times of distress. The same could be said of us, unfortunately, and this caused my mental state to fluctuate and, at times, blood pressure to be high as I lingered on these feelings. However, in the true style of live and let live, I let it go; others did not, but I knew I was the better person and who knows better, does better. I had to. My cancer diary was further influenced through turning the pages of magazines and newspapers and, in later years, twitter, facebook and blogs.

How many of these I read evades me, but they spanned a few years and in doing so, I realised how cancer had really affected not only the rich and the famous, but also ordinary Joe blogs (like me). Prostate cancer is a perennially popular topic and has spawned a massive body of literature, its history engaging all manner of creed and gender. Cancer clearly showed no favouritism and was merciless and scathing in its attack. What nearly all cancer experiences have in common are the similar stories and similar endings. In writing this book, I have learned that writing gathers everything into itself to make a satisfactory piece. My story, my mind acting on the world and the inverse, human anatomy, some or all and more yet unthought-of had to be combined in the right amounts to make this non-fiction book become a reality. I found it increasingly harder to find a flow and continuity of words that inspired me further, and it is not what you write, but how you do it that is crucial for me. This was never about typing for the sake of typing, it was writing about a cancer experience and journey.

The fact that I was ill was something I tried hard not to dwell on; I just got on with living.

An experience such as cancer changed my perspective on life; it gave me the perspective of what things are really truly important in your life. Your family, friends and your spiritual life are all truly important, as is a positive attitude throughout and never giving up. I suppose what concerned me was if and when I came off the current programme due to my body becoming drug resistant, how long it would be before my PSA rose if at all. As we know, drug resistance remains one of the biggest hurdles in cancer treatment. The Stampede Trial Drug programme extended my life through this new advanced treatment, utilising abiraterone and prednisolone. Clearly, these have suited me extremely well, as my body had shown that it was very sensitive and receptive to these drugs.

Recent 2014 figures state that one in two of us will get cancer. It is a disease that will touch every family in the United Kingdom. New drugs are coming onto the market more frequently than at any time before. In an era in which new anti-cancer drugs are used in combination with rotating treatments, hopefully the medical world will be able to stay ahead or at least keep pace with cancer resistance for certain types, enabling a manageable long-term condition for sufferers. I think if you come from a family that cancer has not affected, then the first news hits you harder.

In my family, it has always been around us, hence my initial response when I was diagnosed. Having children helped me greatly, as it gave me the inspiration and will to fight to survive. For me, being a part of the Stampede Trials Drug programme made me feel alive and that I was helping people I did not know or have probably never ever met, regardless of creed, to survive in the future. It is astonishing how my advanced metastatic cancer has been reversed and managed. The outlook seemed bleak at the initial diagnosis stage, but the trial drug programme has lifted that bleakness.

I did not and do not want to spend my remaining time on this earth unwell, as my zest for life has returned. Undergoing a trial programme is hard in lots of ways, as you do not know what to expect, but it seemed to give me the best chance of quality of life in the short term. I was looking for quality of life more than quantity. I was lucky not to develop dangerous side effects to the drugs administered.

My cancer has shrunk and, in some cases, disappeared from areas to which it had spread and I have remained stable for over two and a half years now. That being said, I still have not managed to find anyone to give me non-terminal travel insurance. Life sucks!

One of the most important aspects of my journey was that it was wonderful to have someone (my partner or a family member) with me when there was good news, rather than just supporting me during the bad times. At times during the trials programme, I had lived on the edge, because all the while I acted as a guinea pig, it was a learning curve for the medical world; no one could say what was ahead, since they had never been there before. I hope that my participation will help to change the landscape of those prostate cancer has affected. The war against cancer is far from over, but new weapons like the Stampede Drug Trials programme make for a rosier future.

My mind has gone this way and that these past few years, thanks to all the hospital appointments and other personal things that have gone through my mind. I felt that I could not concentrate fully on any work until all this was over with. What I have found in my cancer journey, though, is that there was a common denominator between cancer diagnosis and treatment. They are more or less the same, but that is where the similarities end.

I marvel at how differently I have coped with what seems to be the same situation.

"I've become institutionalised."

"I just do as I'm told and don't even notice it anymore."

My recovery during January 2015, after my thyroid operation was fuelled by a desire to get my business back into shape and running smoothly. This may not have been the most sensible idea, but when you are under stress, who knows what's sensible anymore. The pressure to work came mostly from myself; every day, I found myself trying and continuing to find a way to exist. I suppose, if I am to be frank, cancer has given me more than it has taken away. Additionally, I was overweight and had type two diabetes when I was diagnosed, but now, I exercise regularly and am attempting to maintain a healthy weight and lifestyle.

In that respect, I believe I am in the best physical shape of my life. Cancer has also made me a more compassionate person; I have found myself readily open and accessible to other cancer sufferers, and freely offer them my advice and time. Spiritually throughout my cancer journey, I found myself mentally in a place of constant questions about my faith that were at times borderline. If I could have just fully believed in my late mother's relationship with God, matters would have been far easier. I don't always understand God, but I believe in Him.

I don't know His name and don't know what religion He would sanction or disavow, but I believe. I don't run around with religious pendants on my chest or Bibles and other holy books under my arm. I don't wake up people by knocking on their doors and pushing magazines in their faces. But I believe. I believe it's all inside me.

My church and sanctuary are all inside my soul. I get dressed up and walk through the aisles of my soul and bow down to my God and pray. I pray for the strength to endure my suffering. I pray for strength and His healing. I have now realised that I'm a stronger believer than many professors of faith.

I was very lucky to have the doctors and nurses I had, especially my Mount Vernon hospital oncologist team. My team painstakingly explained every detail of what I could expect from treatment and never sugar-coated what I was likely to go through during treatment.

Perhaps the most frustrating change for me during my treatment was what affected my sexual life, which was the loss of my libido. The impairment of sexual function was generally unavoidable during my treatment and the extended use of abiraterone, which acted as a chemotherapy agent in tablet form, further compromised my ability to be sexually active.

The substantial adverse physical, mental, psychosocial and economic consequences were what followed, and to some extent still do to this day. I love Grace dearly, but at times, I have felt that I let her down, as my libido has been in decline since April 2012. I do worry so much about neglecting her, as we are only aged 57 and 54. It is not her fidelity that concerns me, more that she is young and obviously has natural needs that I, her partner, am unable to fulfil.

This has become a real-life dilemma for me which I have found extremely hard to accept and talk about to anyone, so quietly, I have suffered.

Survivors of cancer know the stark reality about the life-altering permanent effects with which we likely must contend as a result of our cancer and the ultimate cost of survivorship. Cancer survivorship has three distinct phases: living through, with and beyond cancer. In defining the aforementioned, a survivor is anyone who has been diagnosed with cancer. Survivorship commences at the initial time of disease diagnosis and continues throughout the rest of a patient's life. I have lived through two phases of this survivorship, namely 'through and with.' I have yet to experience the phase of 'living beyond' which, ultimately, is the post-treatment and long-term survivorship phases where the survivor returns to the care of their primary doctor. This is furthered with a long-term health plan care plan about which they have consulted with their oncologist, and then overseen by their primary doctor. I have put my heart and soul into this book and it has become very personal. The whole experience and journey have made me determined to have a productive and meaningful life and, where possible, help other survivors to do the same. I hope and pray you will too. I, by the Grace of God, do. "Smile."

Over the past three years, I have witnessed the deaths of colleagues with whom I have worked. In addition, other male and female colleagues are now walking the cancer pathway, as are close friends' parents who have been diagnosed with the same disease that I have. Fortunately, I have been able to support and talk them through this difficult period in their lives. I feel their pain in so many ways. I know also that I must take a back seat so as not to fall into the trap I have often mentioned, that the level of anxiety one person with cancer experiences may differ from that of another person. Some of these feelings I experienced included being tense, fearful and apprehensive, not to mention finding myself pacing up and down, shaky, jittery, nervous, confused and disoriented. From a personal perspective and contrary to what one might expect, patients with advanced cancer experience anxiety not due to fear of death, but more often from fear of uncontrolled pain, being left alone or dependency on others.

No one can tell you how you should feel about something. Anyone who tries to tell you that how you are feeling is wrong is wrong.

The simplest of daily tasks are becoming easier and some flexibility has returned to certain joints in my body. I continue on with my journey back to wellness with better exercise and nutrition routines; I know now how certain food kinds and beverages make my body feel and it isn't great. I have made a conscious decision not to drink alcohol throughout my cancer treatment. My body was fighting a big enough battle trying to rebuild and didn't need the extra pressures of trying to process alcohol.

It's a big change for me, but alcohol is loaded with sugars and preservatives that are hard to process, and having type two diabetes does not help matters.

It's not been easy, in fact it's been torturously bloody hard, but I know my life now depends on it. I know that the road to wellness is a winding one and only through re-designing it will I survive. As to the future of cancer prevention, if more people follow current medical recommendations for prevention and early detection, then the chances of cancer will ultimately be lessened. By reducing their cancer risk-heightening behaviours such as smoking, bad diets, alcohol use, inactivity and excessive exposure to sunlight, the danger is lessened.

By using available vaccines against cancer-causing viruses, such as hepatitis B and papilloma viruses, and by taking precautionary measures to protect individuals who inherit the several known gene variants that confer significantly increased risks of cancer, the risk is lessened. 'Will I ever fall into remission?' is the primary question, which can only be answered by saying my life is in my hands and my hands only.

To remain standing while so many have fallen is a miracle in itself, and this is echoed every time I attend my clinical appointments and my PSA results are conveyed to me as less than 0.1.

Financially, over the last three and a half years, cancer has impacted me and my family greatly. I have only worked between six and seven weeks during this time. Registered as disabled on benefits made matters worse and the anguish I felt as a result was mentally taxing.

The costs of driving to and from hospital, as well as lengthy expensive parking fees for consultation visits, as well as emergency attendances dug deep into our pockets. A virtual re-fit of my wardrobe was required, as I gained weight due to steroid medication; I began to see why weight lifters used these tablets for training supplements. Saving funds were raided and exhausted in attempts to meet financial obligations, as well as trying to set up a home-based business. However, I was always a field agent and that attempt came to a grinding bumpy halt.

Without Grace steering the household ship, it would have been next to impossible to sustain against this onslaught. My brother Kelly was a godsend as he occasionally propped me up, as was my son Nathan. In some strange way, we ended up overcoming the financial hardship before us. Many a sleepless night was had while I wrestled with dreams of different legal ways to stay afloat as my consultancy business took a nosedive and only through careful manipulation and manoeuvring was I able to save it from crashing. I believe, if you live good with people and treat people right in life, you will be rewarded. It doesn't necessary mean that it is a financial reward, but let's put it this way: the bailiffs never came knocking at our door.

Every story of a cancer survivor is different and deserves to be heard. Being a survivor does not mean I was strong or brave or cured. It was about me embracing and coming to terms with the disease I have.

It's difficult to fully understand what life will be like from here on out, after facing a life-limiting disease and coming back from it. I never realized how important intimacy and human contact were, until I couldn't have them freely anymore. Until my partner, family and friends were afraid to touch me. To you reading this might seem trivial, but to me it was devastating.

It has taken me a long time to realise that life starts again in a different way. I think you do look differently at life, and silly things don't seem to matter anymore. It was perfectly 'normal' that I wasn't the same person I was before. I am now adjusting to my new normal on my own time and anyone who has gone through cancer will, too.

There's no going back to the 'old me'... there's only moving forward to find the 'new me.'

www.ingramcontent.com/pod-product-compliance
Lightning Source LLC
Chambersburg PA
CBHW072123270326
41931CB00010B/1647